IMAGES
of America

DETROIT'S HOSPITALS, HEALERS, AND HELPERS

IMAGES
of America

DETROIT'S HOSPITALS, HEALERS, AND HELPERS

Patricia Ibbotson

ARCADIA
PUBLISHING

ISBN 978-0-7385-3223-3

Published by Arcadia Publishing
Charleston, South Carolina

Printed in the United States of America

Library of Congress Catalog Card Number: 2003114304

For all general information contact Arcadia Publishing at:
Telephone 843-853-2070
Fax 843-853-0044
E-mail sales@arcadiapublishing.com
For customer service and orders:
Toll-Free 1-888-313-2665

Visit us on the Internet at www.arcadiapublishing.com

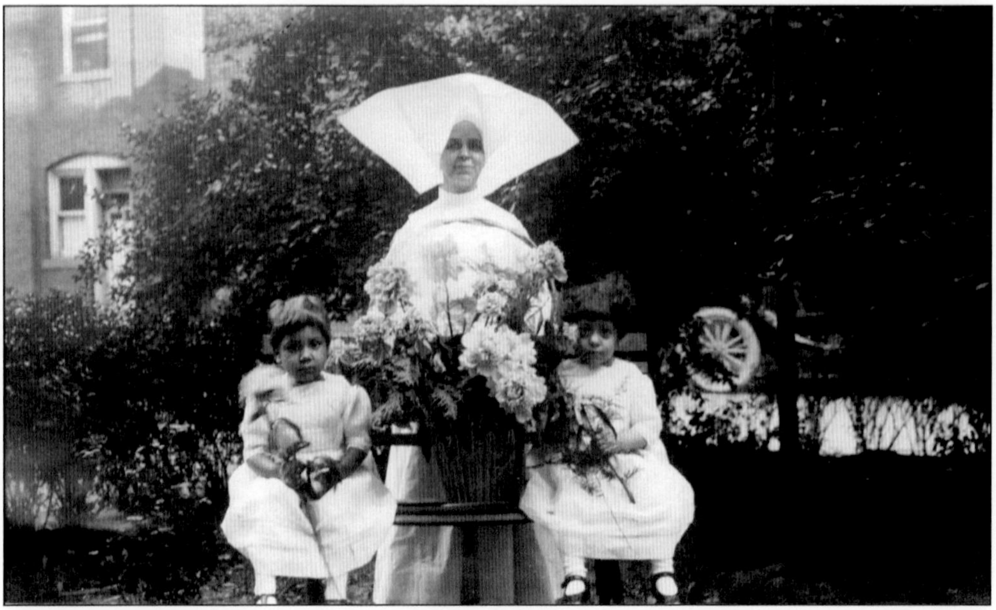

IN THE GARDEN, c. 1926. Sister Redemptoris of the Daughters of Charity is pictured here with two of the children from the House of Providence. (Courtesy Daughter of Charity Archives, Mater Dei Provincialate, Evansville, Indiana.)

Contents

Acknowledgments		6
Introduction		7
1.	In the Beginning	9
2.	Sanitariums and Asylums	45
3.	Eloise	63
4.	The Visiting Nurse Association of Detroit	87
5.	Benevolent Societies	93
6.	Now Just a Memory	107

ACKNOWLEDGMENTS

My special thanks are due to the following people who have contributed in ways great and small to my ability to assemble photographs and information for this book: John Gibson and David Poremba, Burton Historical Collection, Detroit Public Library; Mary J. Wallace, Audiovisual Specialist, Walter P. Reuther Library, Wayne State University; Ernie and Jo Johnson, Friends of Eloise and the Westland Historical Commission; Carol Will, Archivist, Daughters of Charity, Mater Dei Provincialate, Evansville, Indiana; Kirt Gross, Curator of Research, Dearborn Historical Museum; Valerie Latzman and Virginia Presson, Wayne Historical Museum; Roman Godzak, Archivist, Archdiocese of Detroit; Melanie Bazil, Senior Archivist, Henry Ford Health Services, Archives and Historical Collection; Debbie Larsen, Mount Clemens Public Library; Betty Lou Morris, Archivist, Detroit Society for Genealogical Research, Inc.; Sr. Michaeline Lewandowski, archivist, Sisters of Mercy, Farmington, Michigan; Janet Husband; and last, but not least, Cheryl Strange-Laetsch for sharing postcards and assisting in scanning photos.

This book is dedicated to helpers and healers, past and present.

"There is no greater calling than to serve your fellow man."

"There is no greater contribution than to help the weak."

"There is no greater satisfaction than to have done it well."

Walter P. Reuther, 1907–1970

INTRODUCTION

The history of hospitals in Michigan dates back to the care provided to sick men in Michigan's early military garrisons. The log book of Captain Alex Harrison, of the *Gage*, a boat that was unloading at the Detroit wharf, included this story: "October 11, 1785. One hand sent to the hospital October 14. Durett came on board in place of Butler, gone to the hospital." A report of June 24, 1790, describes the garrison hospital as one room equipped with 21 single berths and a single chimney.

All of the hospitals in Michigan, as well as homes for the aged and orphans, evolved from the poorhouse system. By 1832 a poorhouse was established in Hamtramck Township, Wayne County, Michigan, two miles from the Detroit city limits. It was specified in the poor law act of 1829 that the poorhouse directors might admit lunatics and other diseased persons, if the disease were not contagious. The cholera epidemic of 1832 strained the ability of this ramshackle poorhouse to provide even minimal care to the many afflicted, including those orphaned by this devastating epidemic. It was then that 280 acres of land were purchased in Nankin Township by the County of Wayne for the purpose of establishing a poorhouse and farm there. By 1841, this poorhouse also became an asylum for the mentally ill, and it later became the Wayne County House, a place that housed the poor, the old, and the infirm. In 1933 a general hospital was established here, and this complex grew to accommodate 10,000 patients, later becoming Wayne County General Hospital and Infirmary in 1945.

Many Michigan hospitals had their beginnings as institutions founded by religions or religious orders. The first private hospital in Michigan was St. Mary's which was founded as St. Vincent's Hospital June 9, 1845. Although this was a Roman Catholic institution, it was opened as a public hospital and payment for care was originally provided by popular subscription. It was founded by four nuns of the Daughters of Charity, and it took in both the mentally ill and people suffering from infectious diseases. The nuns who founded St. Mary's Hospital also founded several other institutions including the House of Providence (for destitute women and children), Providence Hospital, and The Michigan State Retreat (later called St. Joseph's Retreat). St. Joseph's Mercy Hospital, founded by the Sisters of Mercy, which later operated two branches in greater Michigan, and St. John's Hospital, founded by the Sisters of St. Joseph, are two other well-known Detroit hospitals operated by religious orders.

Religious hospitals were not limited to those of Roman Catholic origins. St. Luke's Hospital and Children's Home, which was operated by St. Paul's Protestant Episcopal Church, was another Detroit hospital under Protestant auspices. Evangelical Deaconess, founded in 1919 by a German Lutheran group, was another Detroit hospital with religious origins. The William Booth Memorial Home and Hospital, run by the Salvation Army, was a maternity hospital. Sinai Hospital was founded to service the Jewish community.

Many hospitals were founded to meet specific needs, such as those to care for contagious diseases, such as tuberculosis, which was the leading cause of death at the turn of the century. Among them are the Detroit Tuberculosis Sanitarium (better known as the William H. Maybury Sanitarium), Herman Kiefer Hospital, Boulevard Sanitarium, and the Eloise Sanitarium. Other communicable diseases that were common were smallpox, cholera, diphtheria, and polio.

The benevolent societies filled the need to care for old people and orphans who had no other resources. These were usually church-based homes. In many cases, children were left here, not necessarily because they were orphans, but because their mothers had to work and the institution was used for room and board. The Visiting Nurse Association of Detroit, founded in 1898, provided care in both clinics and patients' homes.

In addition to providing care to patients, several early hospitals established schools of nursing and other training programs for radiology and laboratory personnel. Before the establishment of these training programs, the patient's family or the doctor's or preacher's wife gave bedside care to patients. In addition to bricks and mortar, the core of early hospitals consisted of the people who founded and staffed them.

The metro Detroit area literally had hundreds of hospitals and nursing homes, and it isn't possible to include all of them in one publication. Included here is a representative sampling which includes the oldest and best known—St. Mary's, Harper, Grace, Providence, Woman's, Children's, and Henry Ford Hospitals—as well as those whose names have long ago been forgotten.

One common denominator is that most of these historic hospitals and institutions are gone now. In most cases their original buildings are gone, left only to the hazy memories of those who knew them and the photographs that preserve them. Sadly, in some cases, the photographs are gone, too.

One

In The Beginning

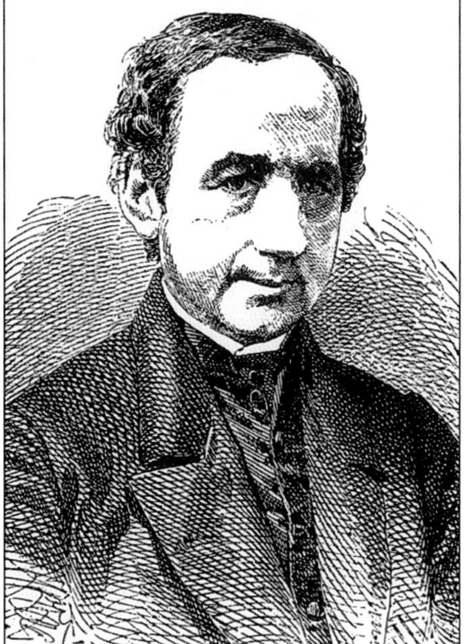

Rev. Martin Kundig
First Superintendent of the Poor
1834-1838

First Superintendent of the Poor. Rev. Martin Kundig ministered to the victims of the cholera epidemic in Detroit and ran the county poorhouse. He also supervised the Wayne County Baths, including the medicinal ones, which were attached to the poorhouse, and the profits arising from the baths were used for charitable purposes. He was described as a giant of a man with a constitution of iron. (Courtesy Eloise Museum, Westland, Michigan.)

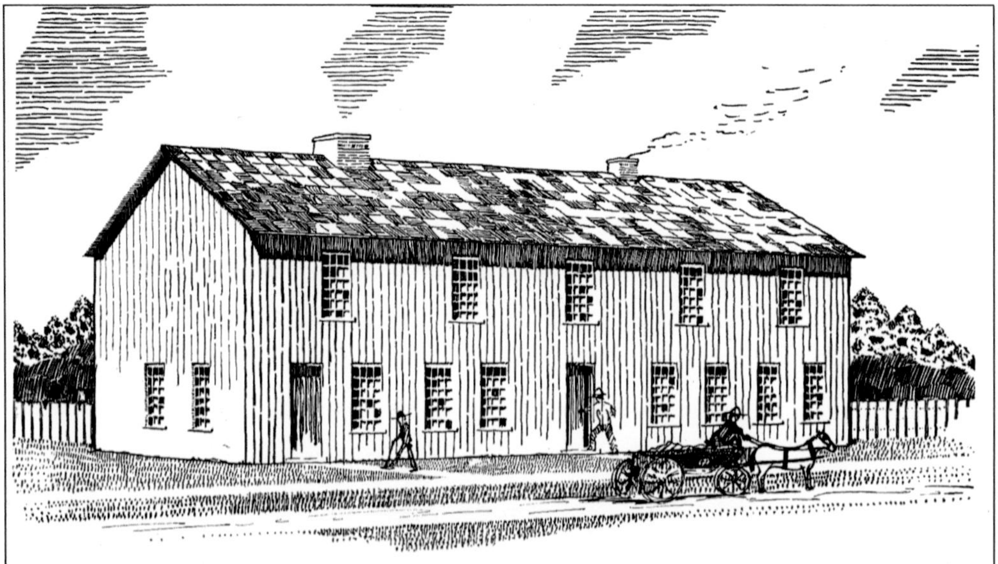

FIRST COUNTY HOUSE, ERECTED IN 1832 IN DETROIT AND USED AS A POOR HOUSE UNTIL 1838

WAYNE COUNTY POORHOUSE, 1838. This wooden building was on the John L. Leib farm on Fort Gratiot Road in Hamtramck Township. The building was 66 feet long, 25 feet wide, and two stories high. The upper floor was divided into six rooms which included two sleeping rooms and two sick rooms—one each for men and women—and two rooms for the superintendent. (Courtesy Eloise Museum, Westland, Michigan.)

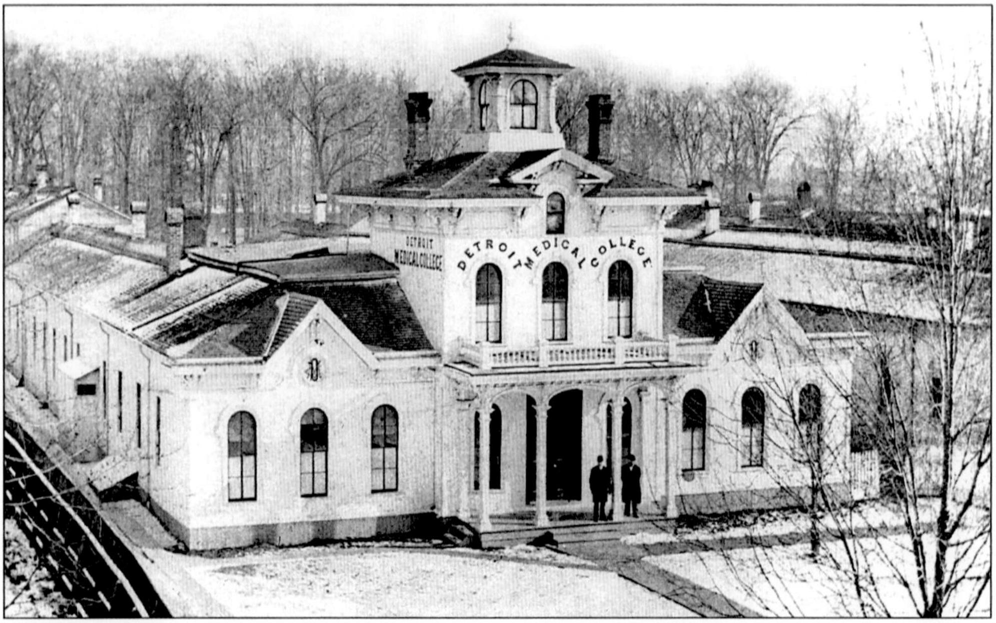

DETROIT MEDICAL COLLEGE, c. 1890. The Detroit Medical College was founded after the Civil War primarily to care for the many ill and disabled soldiers. The demand for doctors was so great that applicants were admitted without regard to their academic credentials, and graduated after two sessions of five months each. Beginning in September 1880, the course was lengthened to three terms of six months each. (Courtesy Walter P. Reuther Library, Wayne State University.)

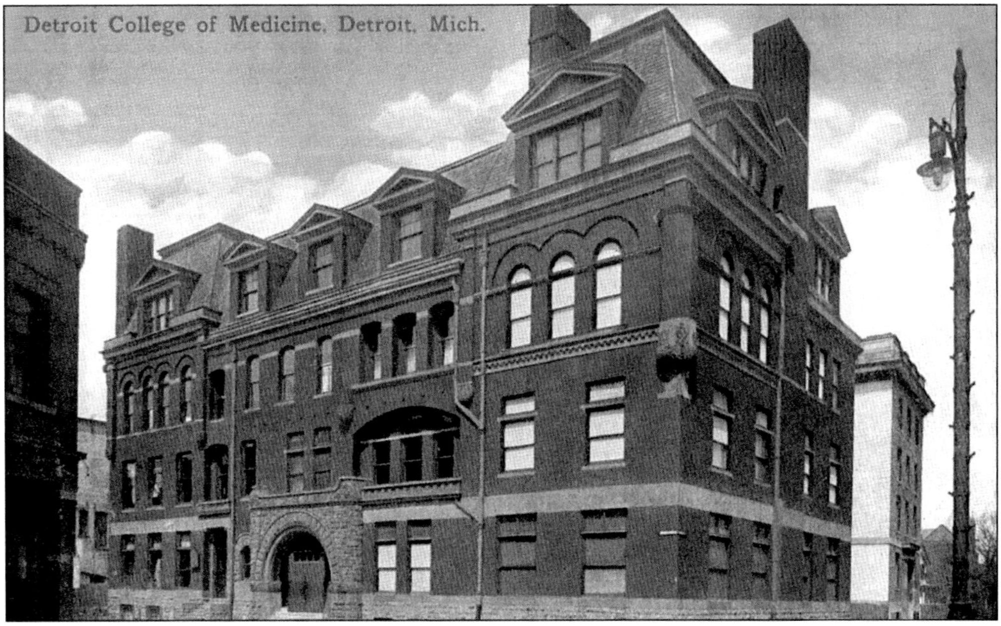

DETROIT COLLEGE OF MEDICINE, c. 1890. This color postcard shows the new headquarters at St. Antoine and Mullett, next to St. Mary's Hospital. The college merged with the Michigan College of Medicine in 1885. It boasted a free ambulance service and a free dispensary. In 1933 this building became Wayne State University's College of Medicine.

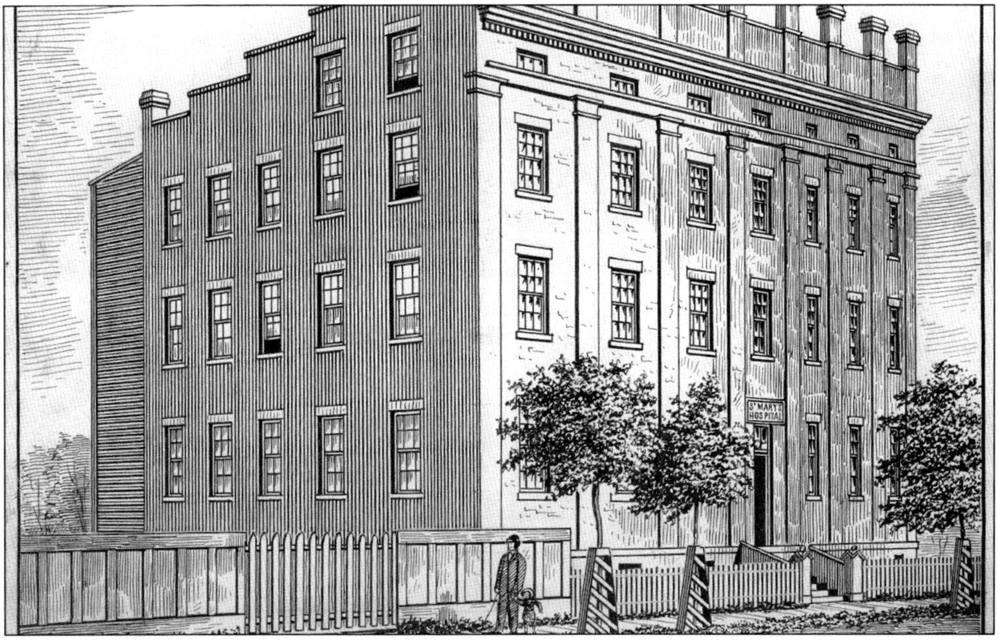

MICHIGAN'S FIRST HOSPITAL, 1850. Founded in 1845 as St. Vincent's Hospital by the Daughters of Charity, St. Mary's was Michigan's first hospital. It provided care to orphans, the insane, and people with contagious diseases and also served, along with Harper Hospital, as the U.S. General Hospital during the Civil War. This was the second hospital building, and it opened November 6, 1850. (Courtesy Burton Historical Collection, Detroit Public Library.)

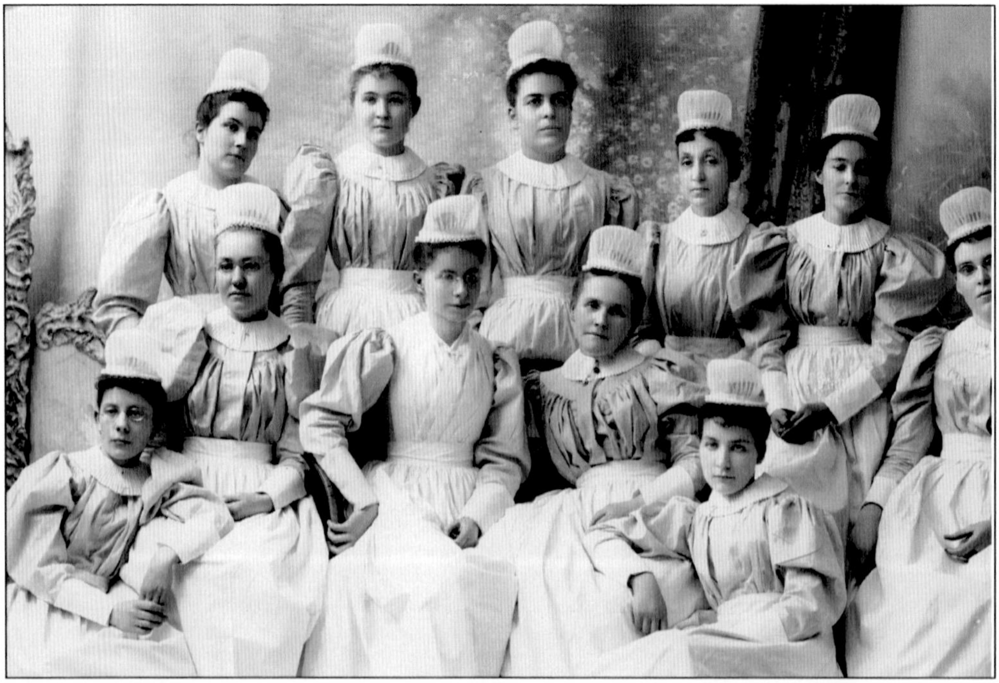

First Graduating Class, St. Mary's Hospital, 1896. Miss Helen Ryan was the superintendent of the nursing school that opened in 1894. Sources say there were 15 graduates, but only 11 are pictured here. (Courtesy Daughters of Charity Archives, Mater Dei Provincialate, Evansville, Indiana.)

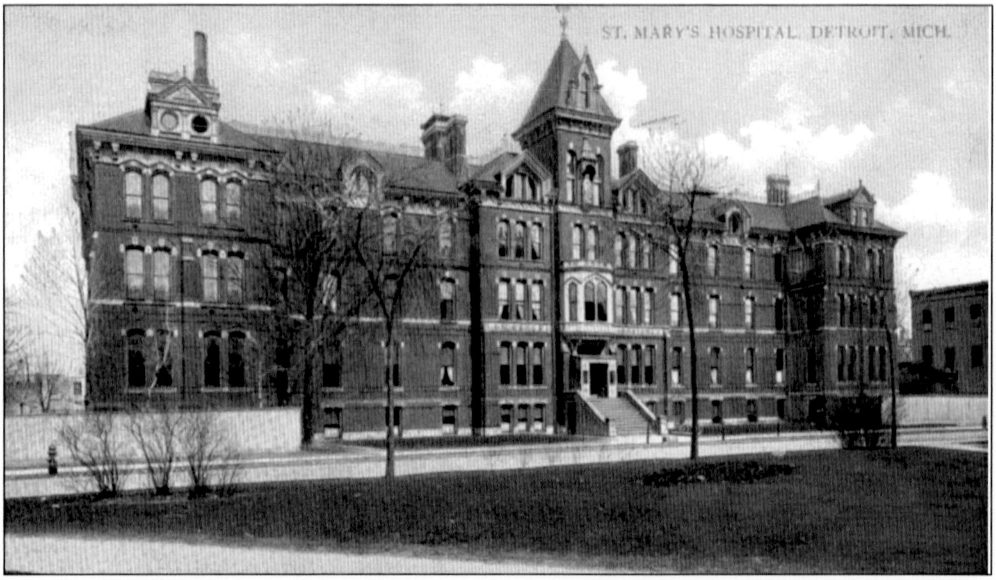

St. Mary's Hospital, 1909. This postcard postmarked May 13, 1909, shows the third edifice built in 1879 which replaced the brick building on St. Antoine Street. This building housed 130 patients, and a free dispensary was maintained in connection to the hospital. St. Mary's provided service to Detroiters for 104 years until it became Detroit Memorial Hospital on December 12, 1949.

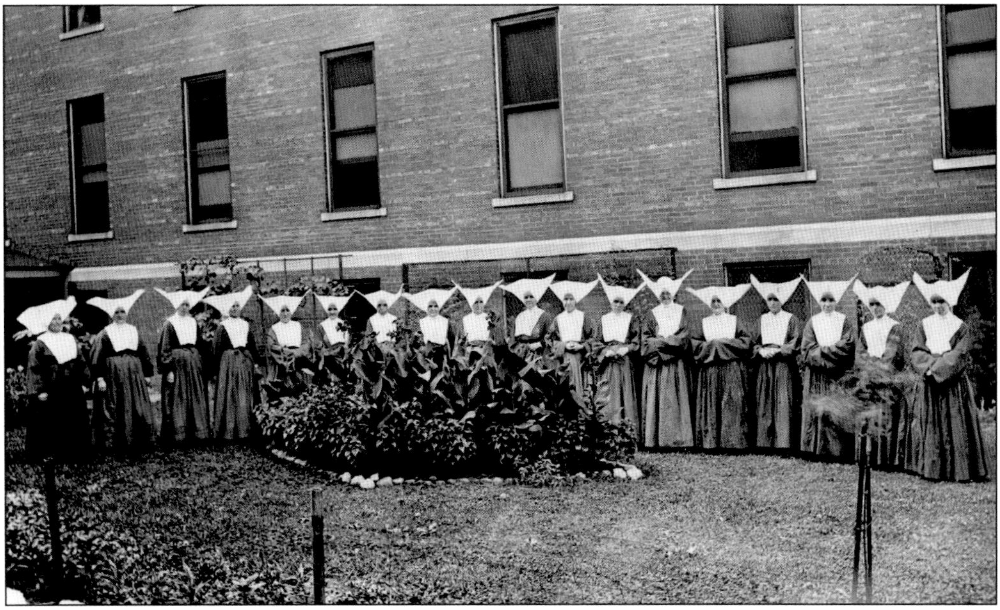

DAUGHTERS OF CHARITY, ST. MARY'S HOSPITAL, c. 1920. Eighteen sisters who staffed St. Mary's are posed in the gardens on the side of the hospital. The Daughters of Charity were easily recognized by their distinctive head pieces. (Courtesy Daughters of Charity Archives, Mater Dei Provincialate, Evansville, Indiana.)

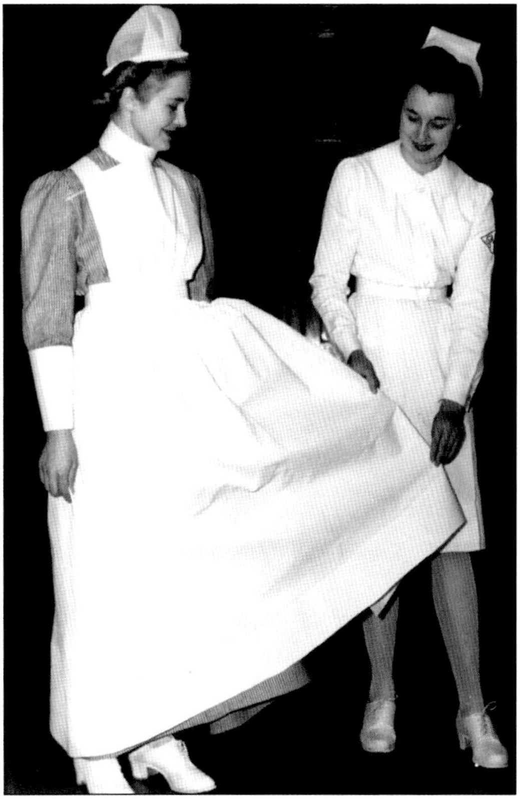

THEN AND NOW: THE 100TH ANNIVERSARY OF ST. MARY'S HOSPITAL, 1945. A nurse in her then-modern 1940s St. Mary's uniform admires the 1890s apparel modeled by a colleague. Nowadays the nurse would be wearing scrubs and running shoes. (Courtesy Burton Historical Collection, Detroit Public Library.)

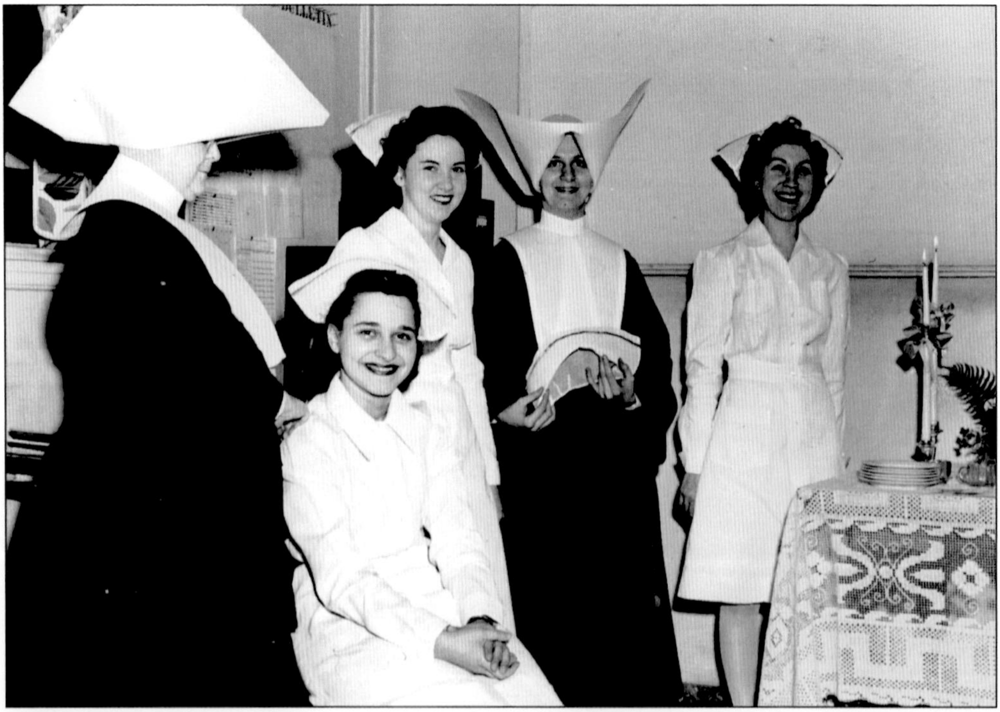

GRADUATION PARTY, ST. MARY'S HOSPITAL, c. 1947. Three smiling graduates of the hospital's three-year nursing program proudly pose with two Daughters of Charity. (Courtesy Daughters of Charity Archives, Mater Dei Provincialate, Evansville, Indiana.)

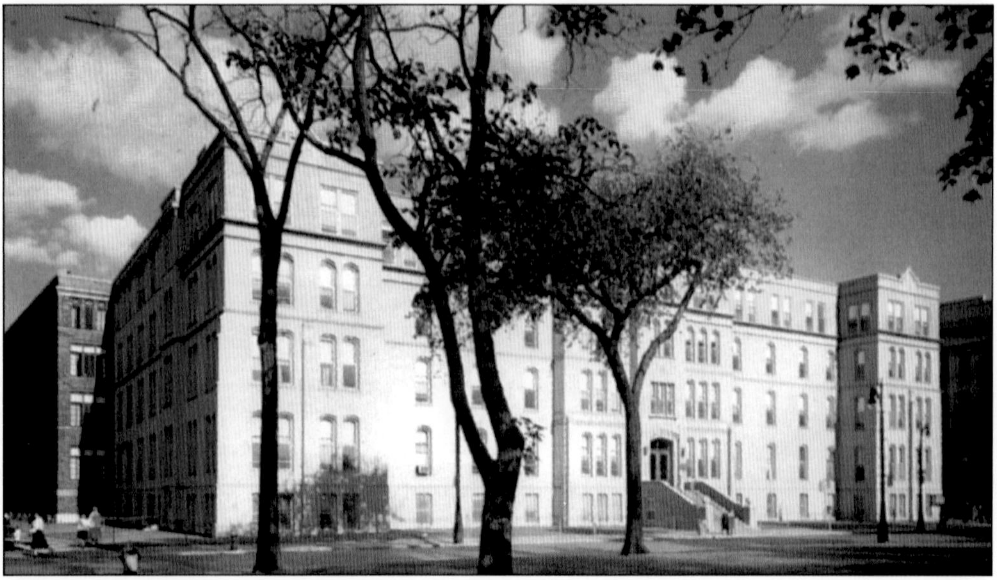

DETROIT MEMORIAL HOSPITAL, 1964. St. Mary's Hospital was extensively modernized over the years, and this is how it looked as Detroit Memorial Hospital. A corporation of St. Mary's physicians purchased and renamed the hospital. This photograph was taken from a hospital calendar for the year 1964. The hospital closed in 1987. A historic marker was placed on this site in 1974, but even the marker is now gone.

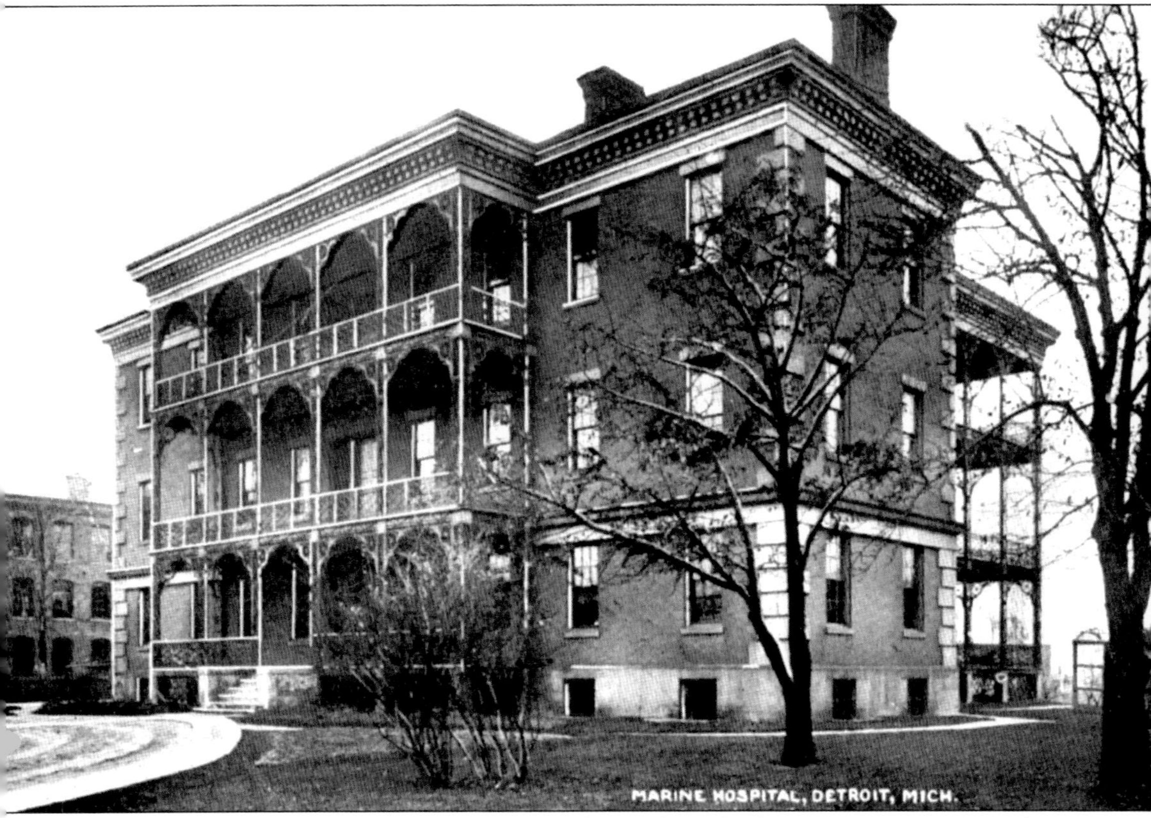

MARINE HOSPITAL, c. 1910. The first marine hospital was built in Detroit in 1857 and it fronted on the Detroit River off Jefferson Avenue. There were roomy verandas with decorative scroll work both in the front and rear of the building. The first 20 patients were transferred from St. Mary's Hospital. The hospital was supported with a tax of 40¢ per month for each person employed on any registered vessel. This fee was deducted from the seamen's wages by the Captain. Any sailor needing medical attention who had been sailing for three months preceding his application for admission could get free care.

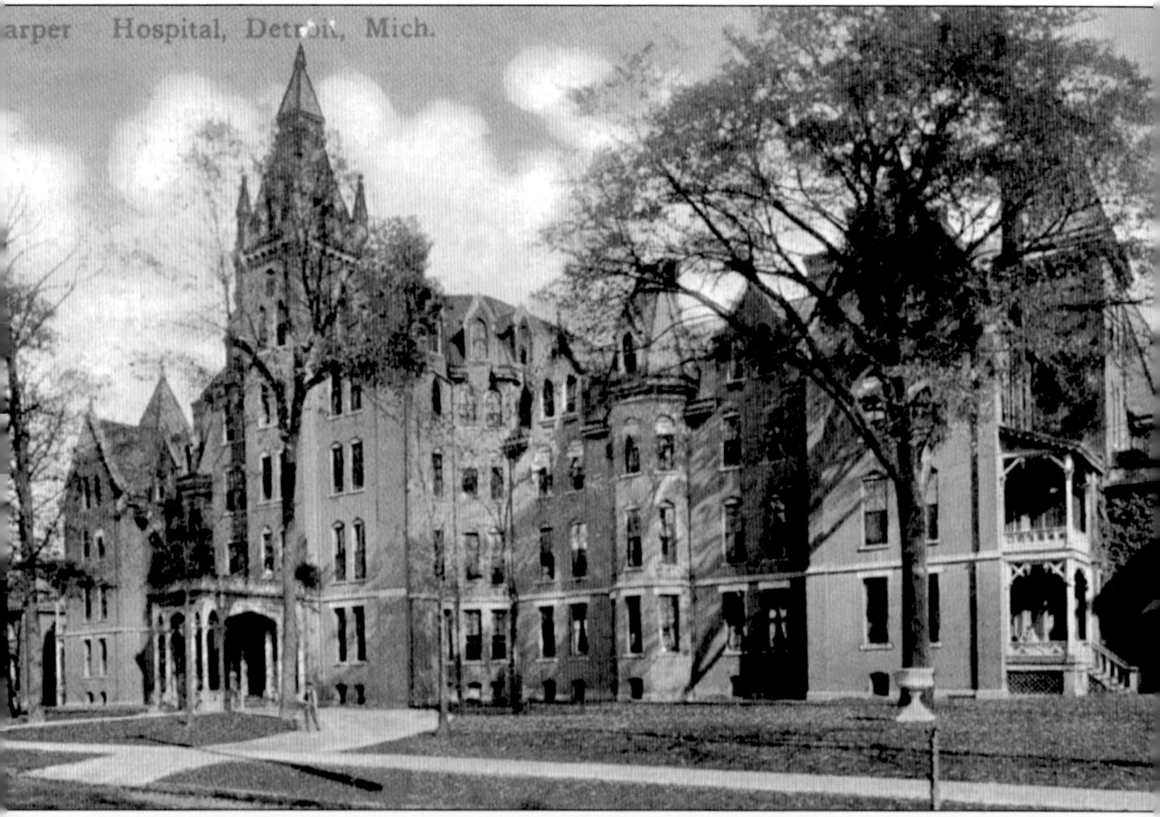

HARPER HOSPITAL, c. 1911. This is one of Detroit's oldest and best known hospitals. It was founded in 1863 and first served, along with St. Mary's Hospital, as the U.S. General Hospital, treating sick and wounded Union soldiers. It was built from land and funds donated by Walter Harper, a wealthy resident of Philadelphia who came to Detroit c. 1832, and his housekeeper/companion, Mrs. Nancy (Ann) Martin. It opened to serve the general public in 1866. Mr. Harper died in 1867, and Mrs. Martin lived in Harper Hospital until the end of her life. This building, shown on a color postcard, opened to patients on June 19, 1884.

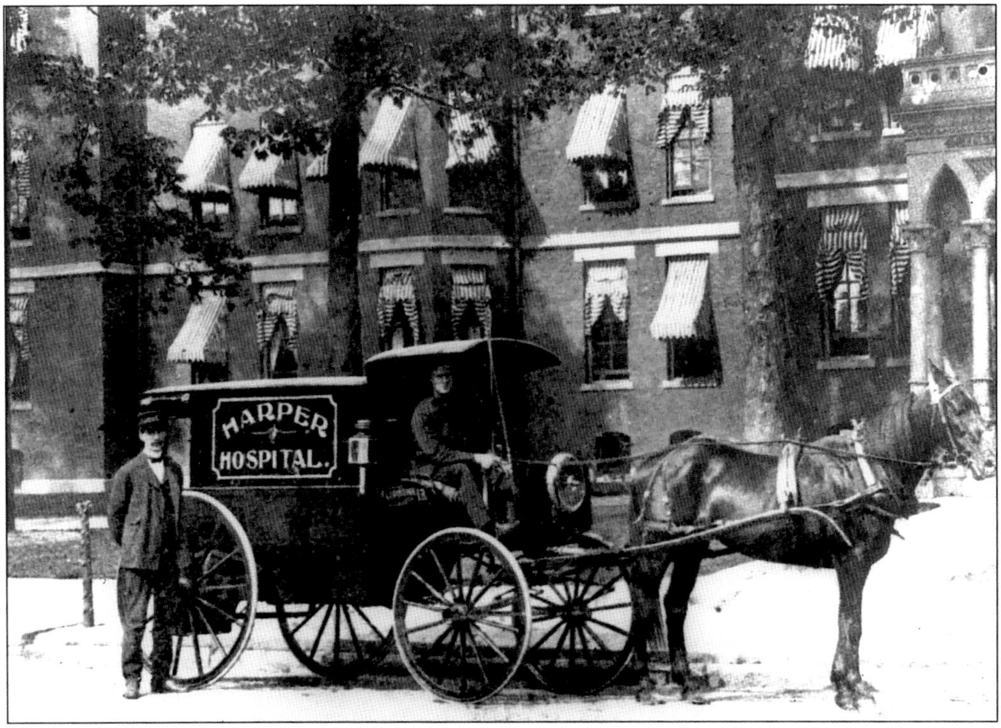

AMBULANCE, HARPER HOSPITAL, 1890. These men are posed with the horse-drawn ambulance in front of Harper Hospital, located at 500 (later 3800) John R. Street. The hospital advertised that the ambulance would meet patients at the train or boat if due notice was sent to the superintendent. In a true emergency, it may have been faster to walk. (Courtesy Walter P. Reuther Library, Wayne State University.)

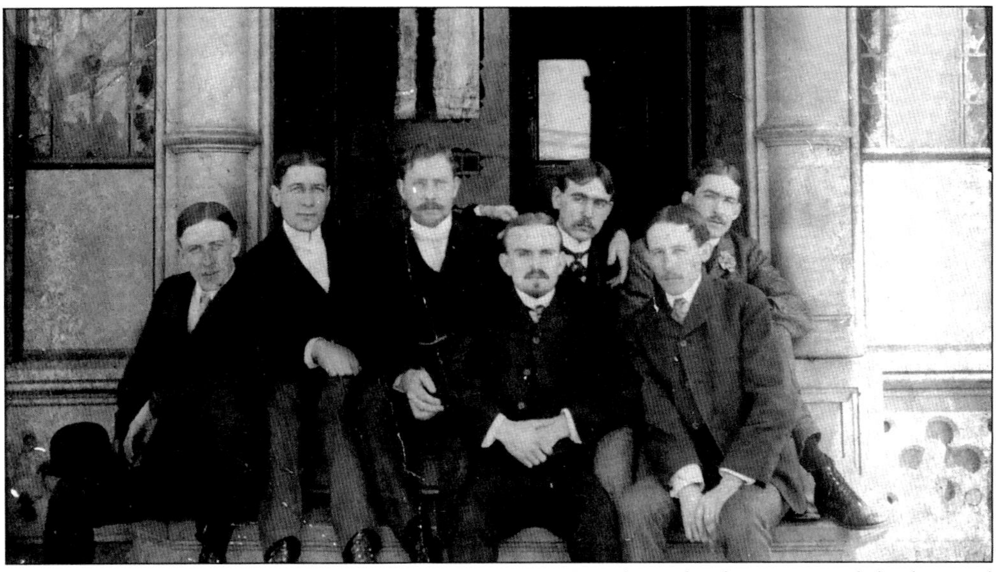

RESIDENT STAFF, HARPER HOSPITAL, 1900–1901. Posed on the front steps of the hospital are seven interns and residents identified only as McDonald, Butler, Mason, Heavenrich, Anderson, and Lewrig. (Courtesy Walter P. Reuther Library, Wayne State University.)

RATES:

Private Rooms, - $10.00 to $21.00 per week.
Wards - - - $7.00 per week.

These rates include Board, plain Washing and Medicine.

All patients are cared for day and night by Trained Nurses.

Special Nurses, devoting their entire time to the patient, furnished at $15.00 per week.

All beds in wards, as well as private rooms, have electric bells communicating with the nurse in charge of hall.

Patients occupying private rooms can be entirely exclusive, and enjoy all the comforts pertaining thereto. They also have the privilege of selecting any reputable physician or surgeon they may choose, but they are expected to pay extra for their services.

All patients are expected to pay in advance. Should they leave before expiration of time paid for, the balance will be refunded.

Cases of emergency received at any time, day or night.

The Hospital's ambulance will meet patients at train or boat if due notice is sent to the Superintendent.

For further particulars address

A. W. SHAW, Superintendent.

HARPER HOSPITAL ROOM RATES AND SERVICES. This is an early advertisement touting the advantages of Harper Hospital. At the turn of the century, patients had private duty nurses, but were expected to pay in advance. (Courtesy Walter P. Reuther Library, Wayne State University.)

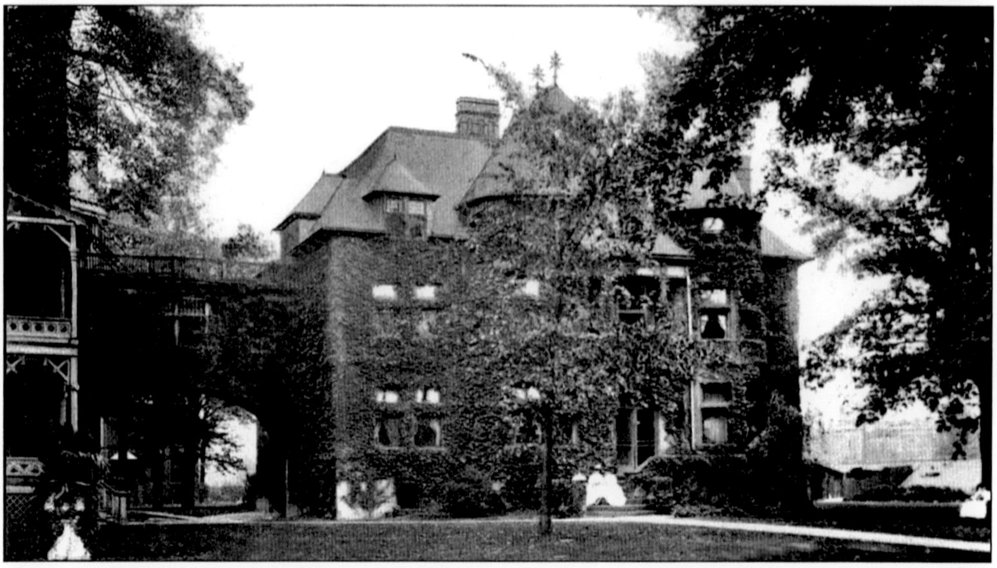

NURSES' HOME, HARPER HOSPITAL. This is a color postcard of the Swain Home. The Richmond Terrace was another residence directly opposite the hospital; together they housed 150 nurses. According to a brochure from the Farrand Training School, these homes were thoroughly equipped and modern in detail, and had reading and reception rooms.

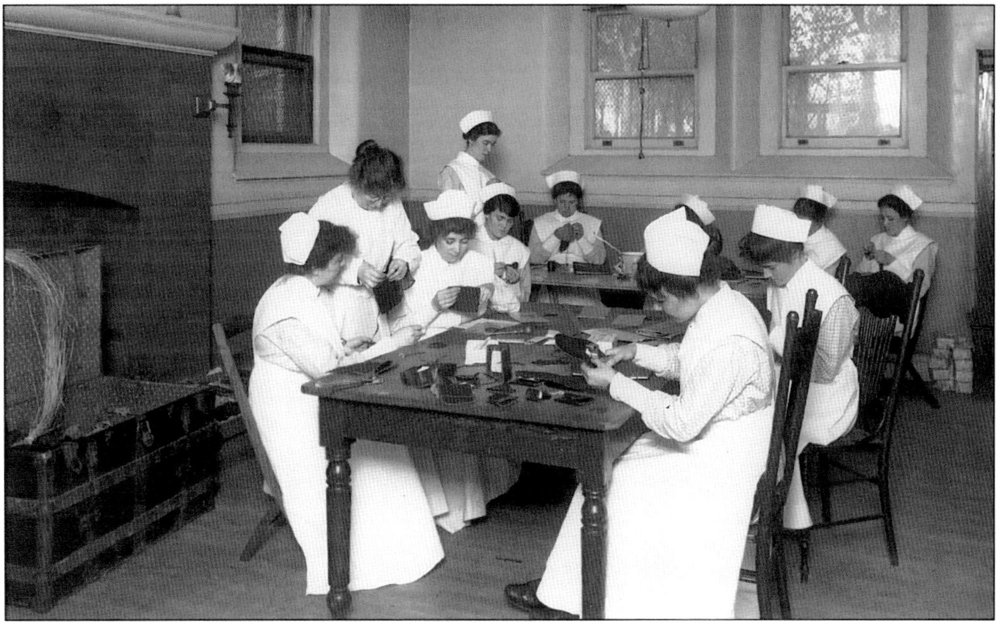

NURSES' CLASS, HARPER HOSPITAL, c. 1910. In this undated photo, Harper Hospital student nurses are working on crafts, and are possibly making wallets. The students wore a distinctive gray and white checked uniform covered by a starched white bib apron which identified them as Harper students. (Courtesy Walter P. Reuther Library, Wayne State University.)

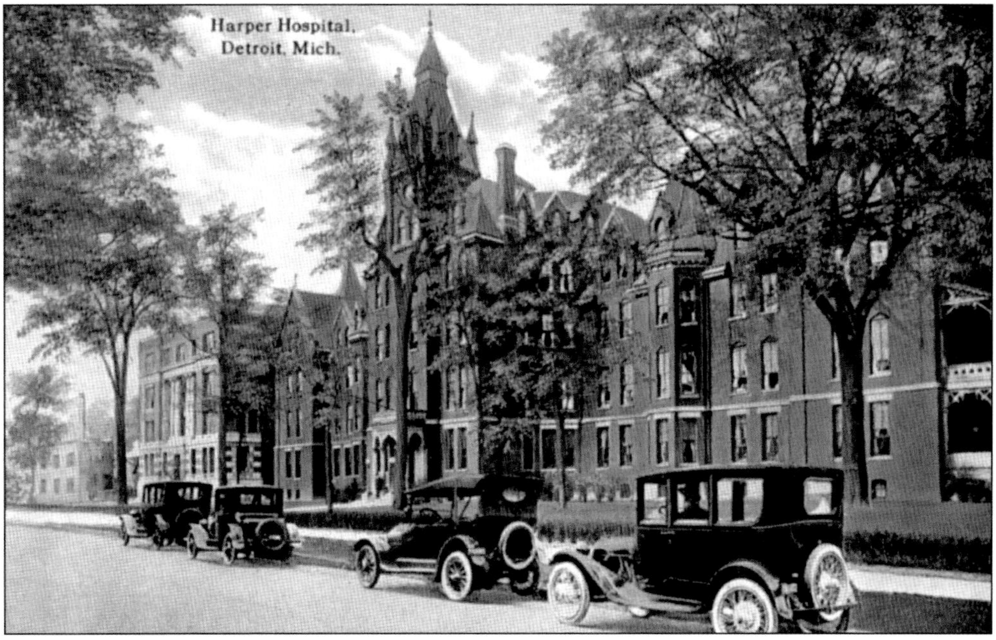

HARPER HOSPITAL, 1920S. The hospital is shown in a slightly different angle in this rare color postcard. For many years, Harper was considered the best hospital in Detroit. Mrs. Henry Ford was a patient there for four weeks in 1907, and her room cost $21 per week. The ambulance charge was $2 and the charge for champagne was $1.55. Her total bill, including board for the nurses, was $118.55.

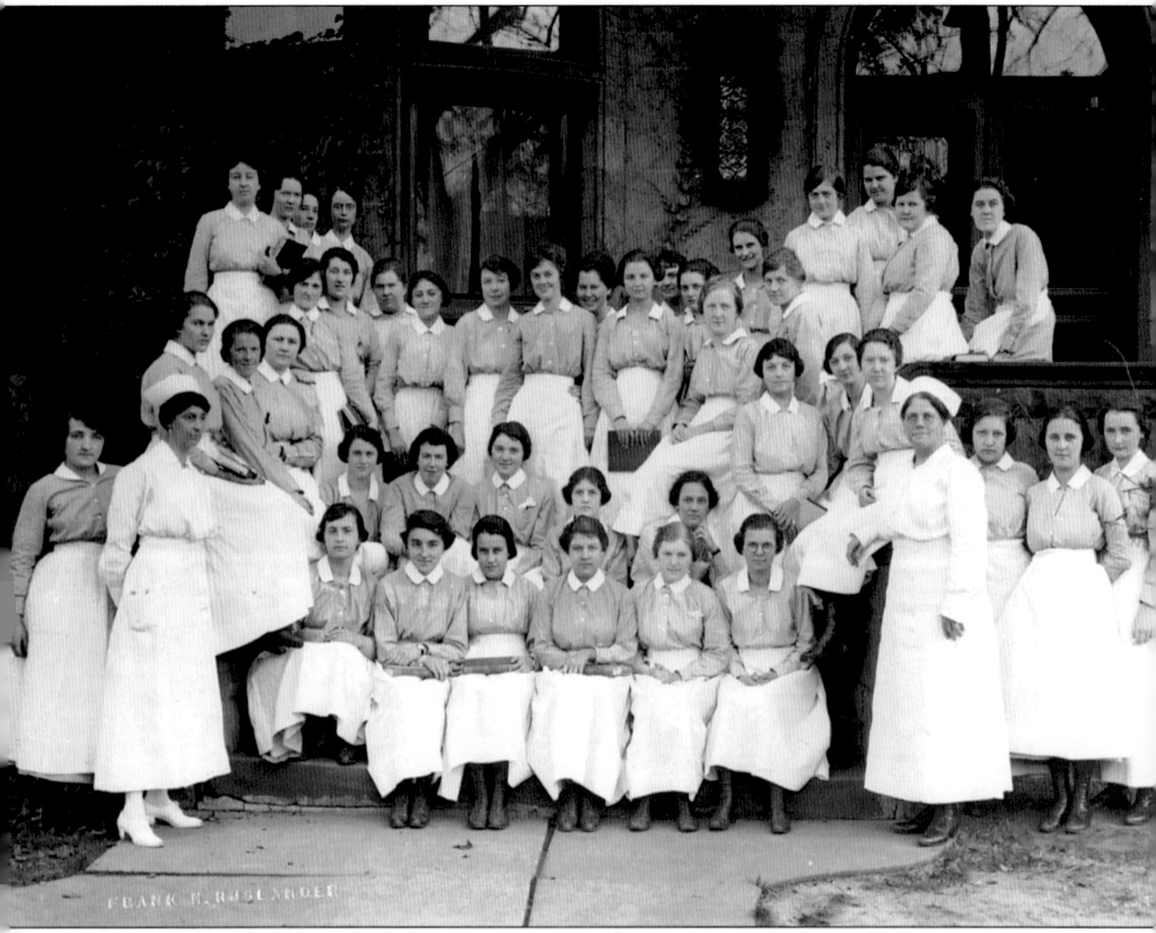

HARPER HOSPITAL, STUDENT NURSE CLASS, 1921. These ladies are probationers of the Farrand Training School for Nurses which was established in 1884 in memory of David Osborn Farrand, M.D. Three classes were formed yearly with students entering in January, April, and September. The students were on probation for three months of their three-year training program. They received their board, a reasonable amount of laundry work, and their uniforms and shoes. Students were not allowed to wear their uniforms in public places. Candidates for the nursing school had to have at least two years of high school or its equivalent, and women of "superior culture" were preferred. Requirements for admission included a letter of reference from a clergyman testifying to good moral character, as well as personal and educational qualifications. (Courtesy Walter P. Reuther Library, Wayne State University.)

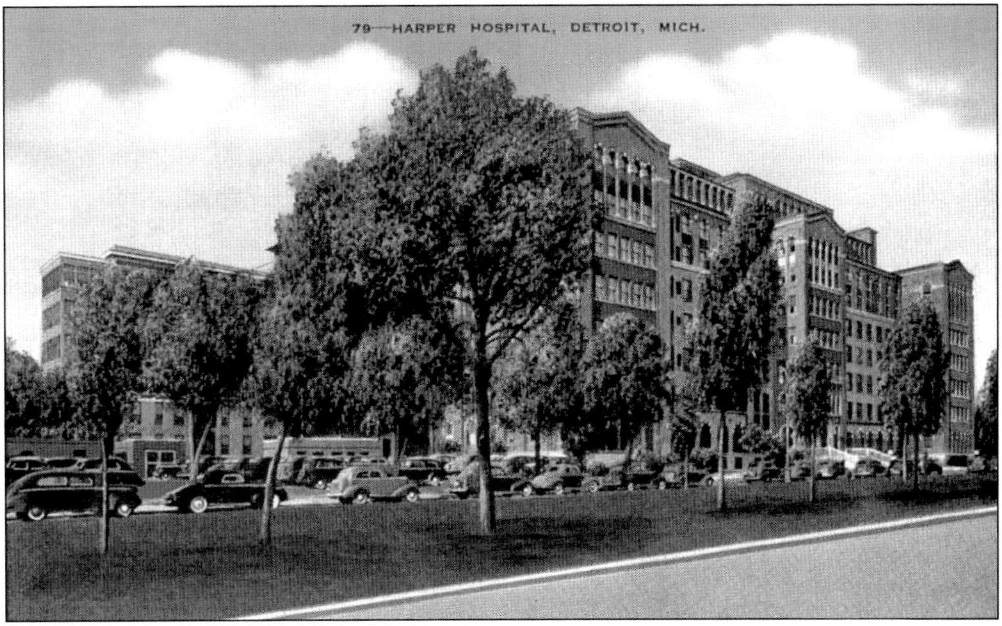

HARPER HOSPITAL, 1940S. Here is a view of a larger hospital built in 1928 which is also on a color postcard. It was located at 3825 Brush Street. The reverse side of the postcard says that Detroit was rated as one of the top three cities in the U.S. for health. Harper Hospital merged with Grace Hospital in 1973. This building was torn down after that.

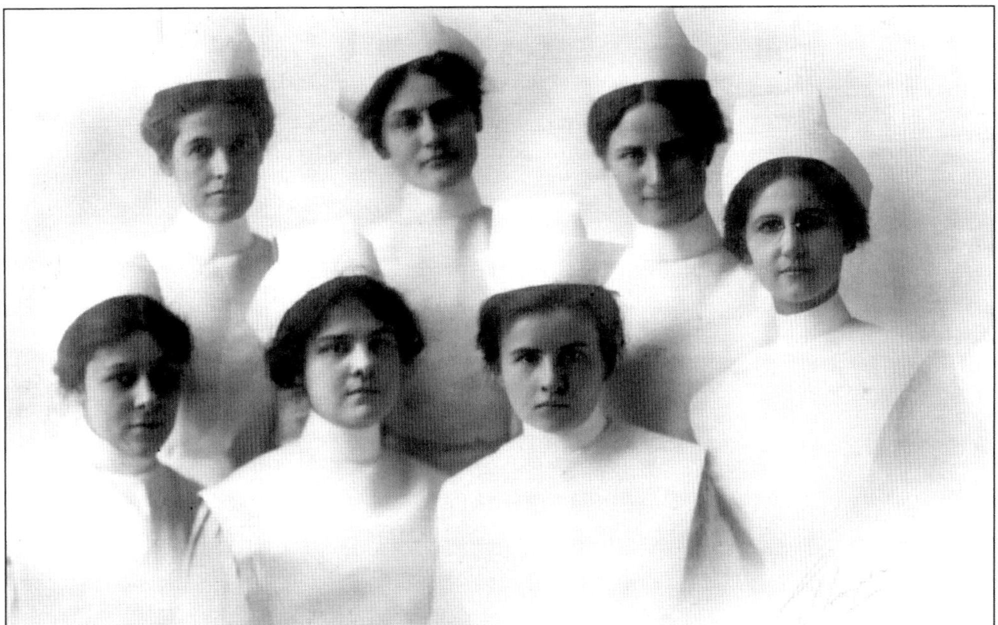

PROVIDENCE HOSPITAL SCHOOL OF NURSING, CLASS OF 1915. Providence started their three-year diploma nursing school in 1910. The seven nurses in this graduating class are, from left to right: (top row) Sarah McLean, Anna Swetish, Marguerite Byrne, and Edith Tovatt; (bottom row) Catherine Miltner, Della Brody, and Elizabeth Becker. (Courtesy Daughters of Charity Archives, Mater Dei Provincialate, Evansville, Indiana.)

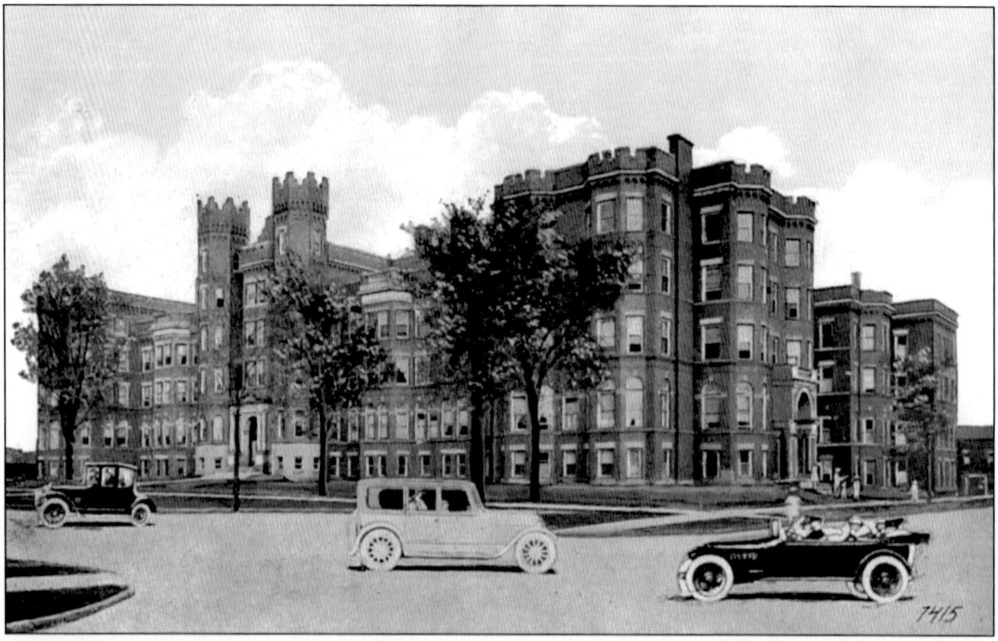

PROVIDENCE HOSPITAL, 1926. This postcard shows the 375-bed general hospital located at 2500 West Grand Boulevard at Fourteenth Street. This hospital evolved from the House of Providence, and it was also founded by the Daughters of Charity. The sister in charge in 1926 was Sister Mary Olympia. The hospital moved from Detroit to Southfield in 1965.

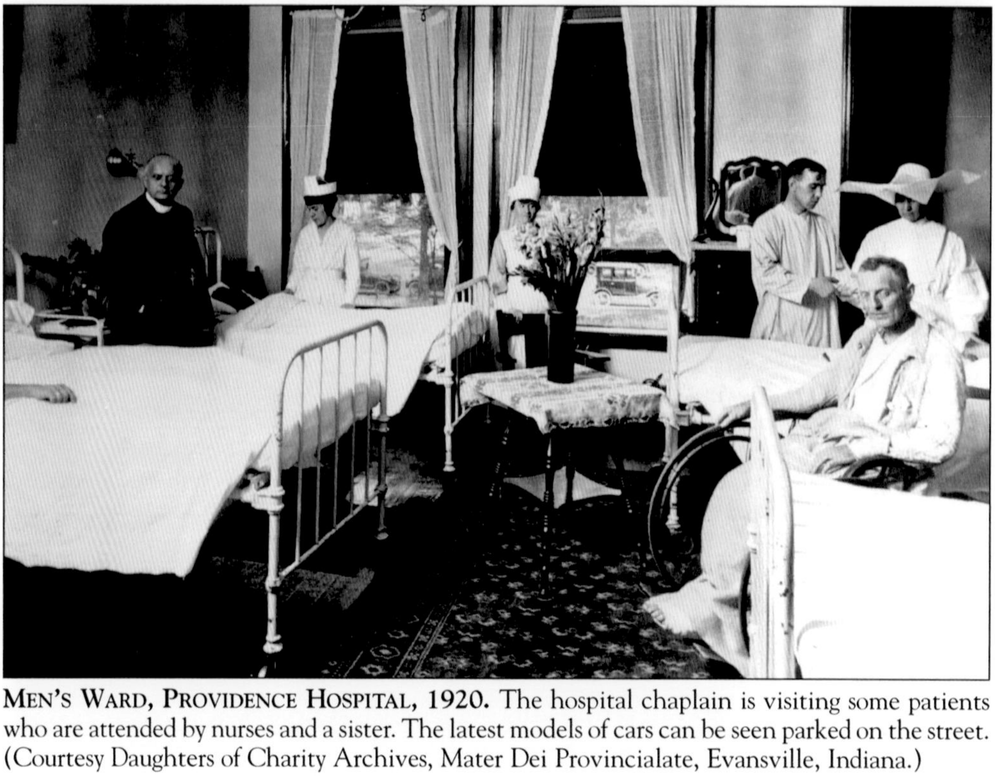

MEN'S WARD, PROVIDENCE HOSPITAL, 1920. The hospital chaplain is visiting some patients who are attended by nurses and a sister. The latest models of cars can be seen parked on the street. (Courtesy Daughters of Charity Archives, Mater Dei Provincialate, Evansville, Indiana.)

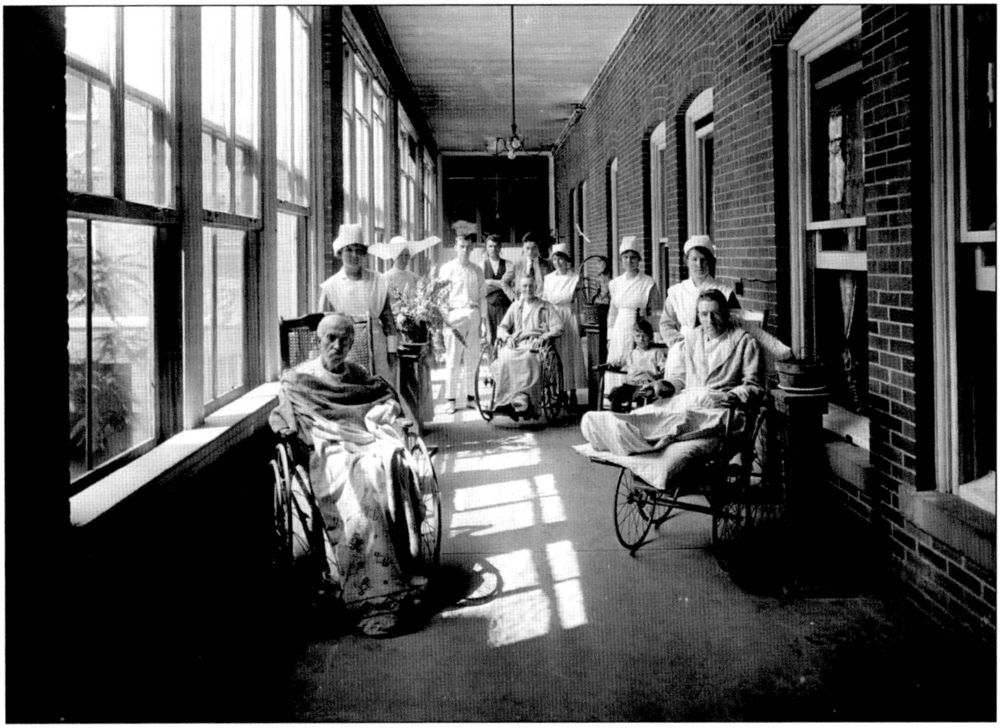

SOLARIUM, PROVIDENCE HOSPITAL, c. 1925. Some patients, including a young boy, are getting some sunshine and a breath of fresh air in this delightful photograph with their nurses and a sister. (Courtesy Daughters of Charity Archives, Mater Dei Provincialate, Evansville, Indiana.)

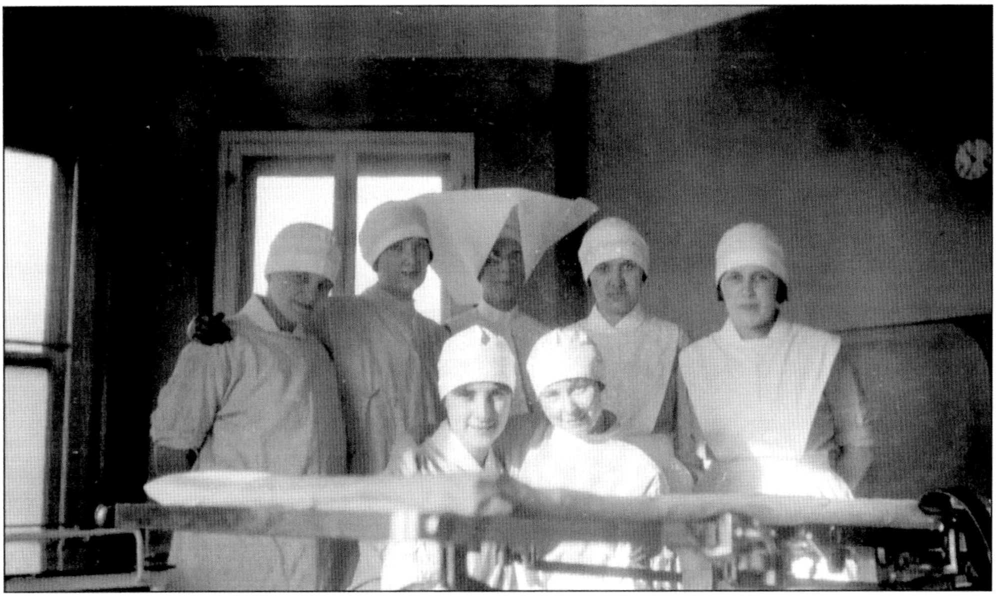

SOME STUDENT NURSES IN THE OPERATING ROOM, PROVIDENCE HOSPITAL, 1920S. Posed behind the operating room table are, from left to right: Freda Verlove, Frances McCartney, Sr. Mary Vincent, Lila Amstertz, Alice Carey, Mary Castlestone, and Stella Flanagan. (Courtesy Daughters of Charity Archives, Mater Dei Provincialate, Evansville, Indiana.)

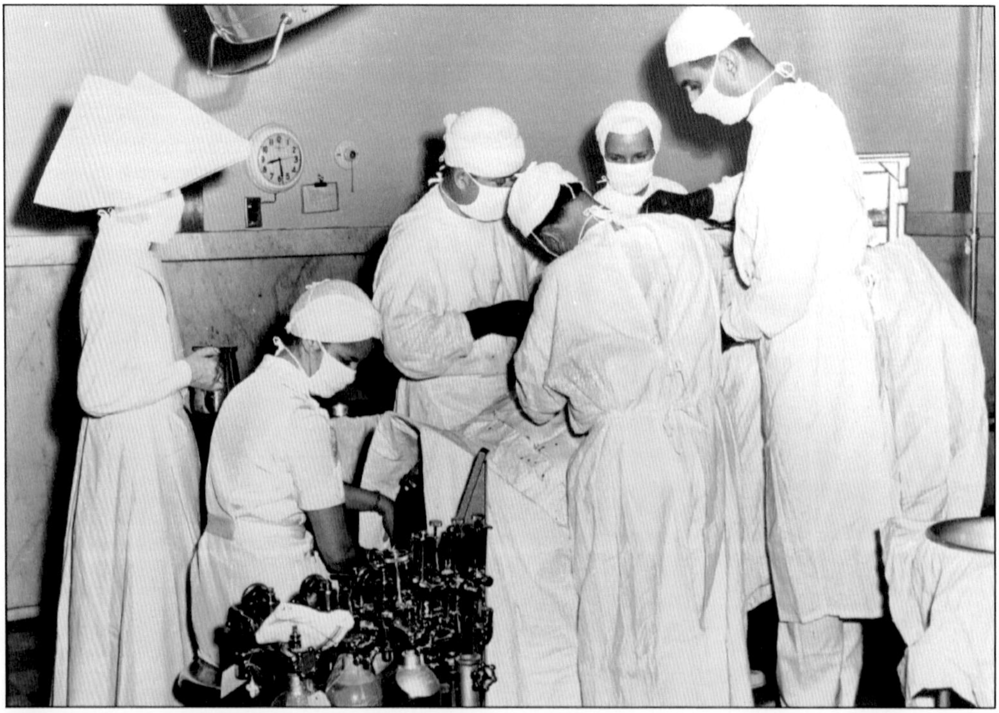

OPERATING ROOM, PROVIDENCE HOSPITAL, c. 1960. In this operating room scene of more than 40 years ago, the circulating nurse (holding the pitcher of water) is a Daughter of Charity sister. (Courtesy Daughters of Charity Archives, Mater Dei Provincialate, Evansville, Indiana.)

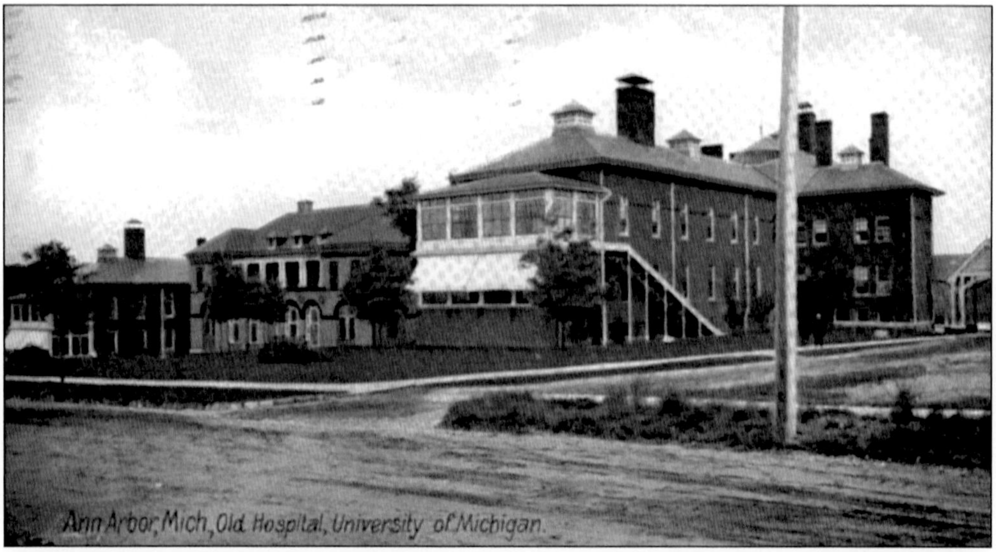

OLD HOSPITAL, UNIVERSITY OF MICHIGAN, ANN ARBOR, 1908. Another early Michigan hospital was the University of Michigan Hospital which opened in 1869. It was the first university-owned hospital in the United States. The first hospital was very small, and it lacked both operating and examining rooms. It was enlarged in 1876 by adding a series of wooden buildings, as shown in this penny postcard which was addressed to Mrs. L.G. Sherman of Kinderhook, Michigan.

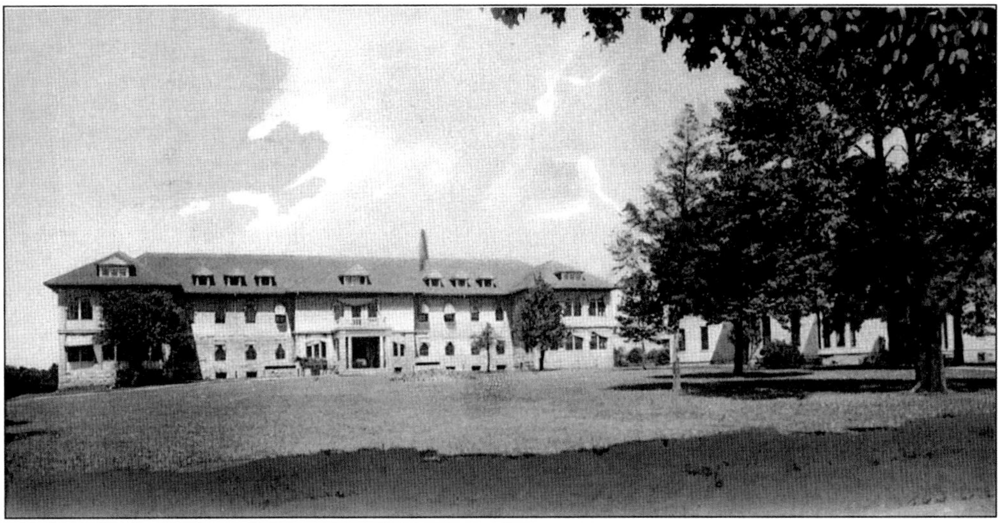

HOMEOPATHIC HOSPITAL AND NURSES HOME, ANN ARBOR, 1909. Homeopathy is a natural system of medicine that utilizes natural plant, animal, or mineral sources in treatment. In 1871 there were over 300 homeopathic physicians in Michigan, and they urged U of M to secure a department to teach homeopathy. This hospital was built in 1899 as part of the University of Michigan hospital complex, and it closed in 1920. It is now the sub-basement of North Hall.

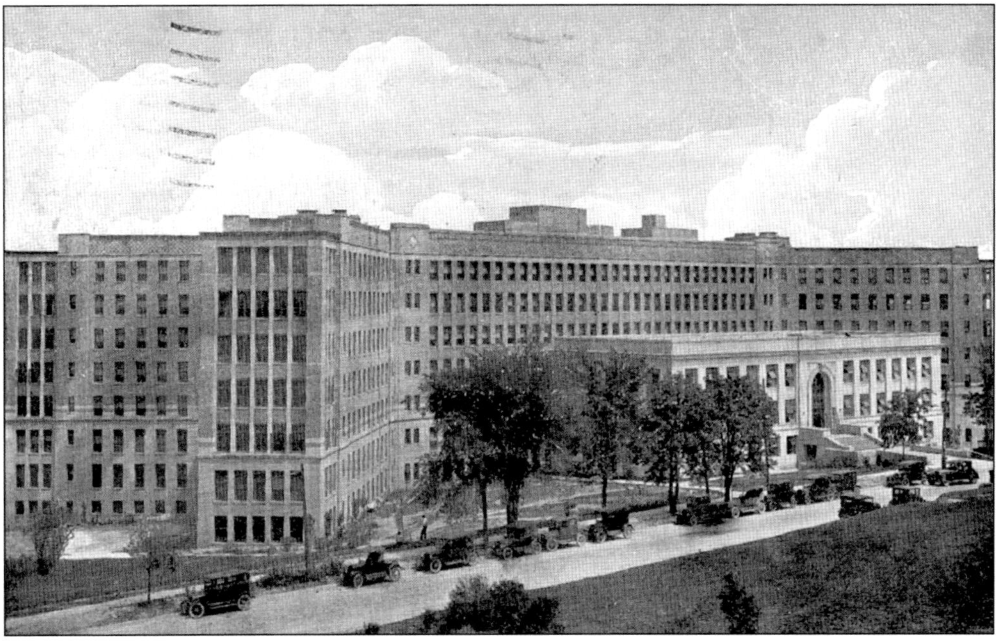

UNIVERSITY OF MICHIGAN HOSPITAL, ANN ARBOR, 1927. This was a state-owned, 1,110-bed hospital in 1927, with only 35 resident physicians and 32 interns. It also had a nursing program which was established in 1891. This building was called Old Main. U of M Hospital is now one of the largest health care complexes in the world, and is ranked among the top ten hospitals in the U.S.

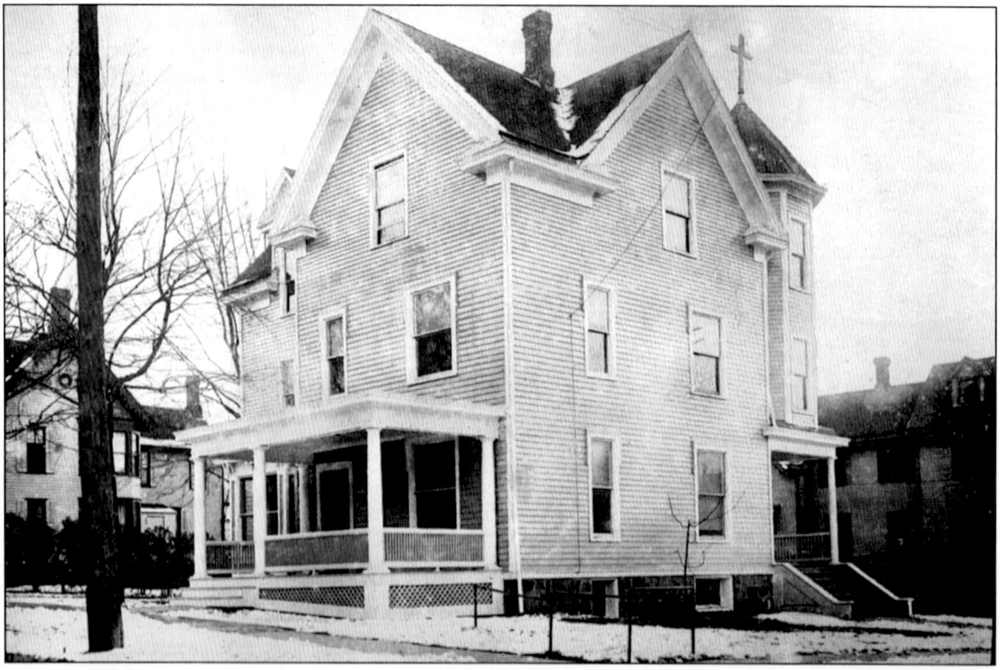

St. Joseph's Sanitarium, Ann Arbor, 1911. What is now a 341-acre hospital complex started out as a 17-bed hospital in Ann Arbor in what had been a private residence. It was founded by the Sisters of Mercy. (Courtesy Sisters of Mercy Archives, Farmington, Michigan.)

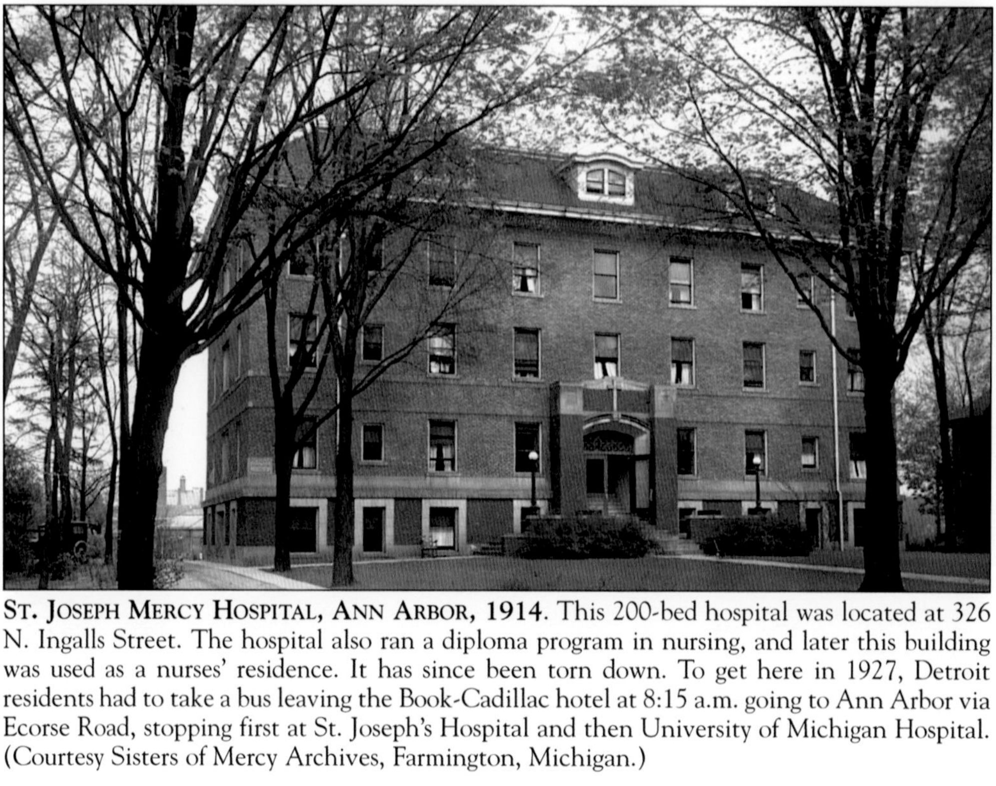

St. Joseph Mercy Hospital, Ann Arbor, 1914. This 200-bed hospital was located at 326 N. Ingalls Street. The hospital also ran a diploma program in nursing, and later this building was used as a nurses' residence. It has since been torn down. To get here in 1927, Detroit residents had to take a bus leaving the Book-Cadillac hotel at 8:15 a.m. going to Ann Arbor via Ecorse Road, stopping first at St. Joseph's Hospital and then University of Michigan Hospital. (Courtesy Sisters of Mercy Archives, Farmington, Michigan.)

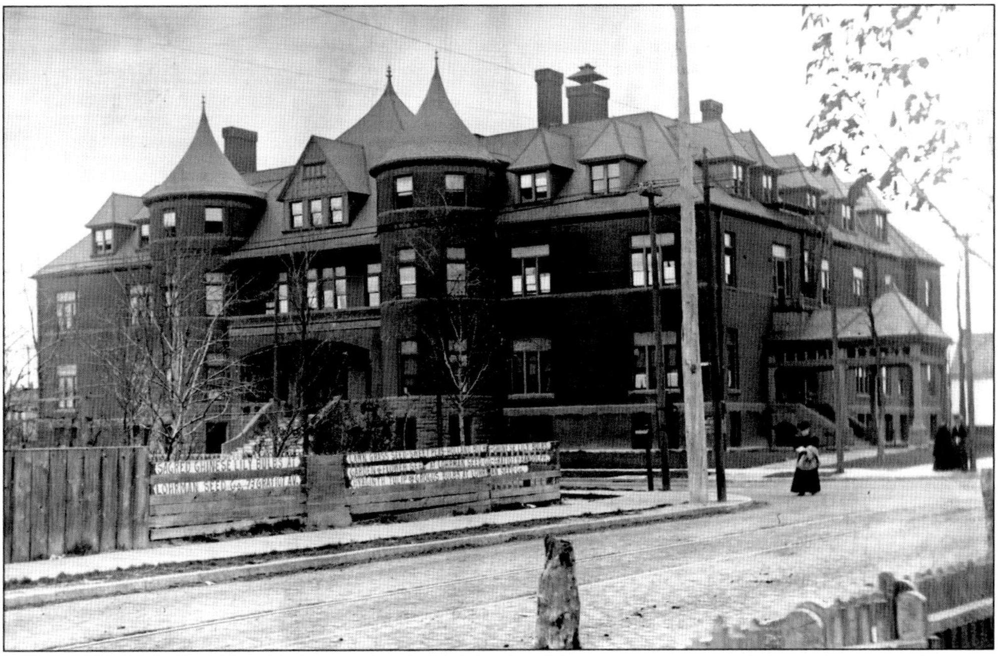

WOMAN'S HOSPITAL, FIRST BUILDING. This early Detroit hospital was founded in 1869 to provide care and shelter to abandoned, widowed, and unwed mothers and their babies. It had its start in November 1868 when seven members of the Ladies' Christian Union opened the Woman's Hospital and Foundling's Home in a tenement at Cass Avenue and Montcalm. The entire staff and Board of Trustees of this hospital were women. (Courtesy Burton Historical Collection, Detroit Public Library.)

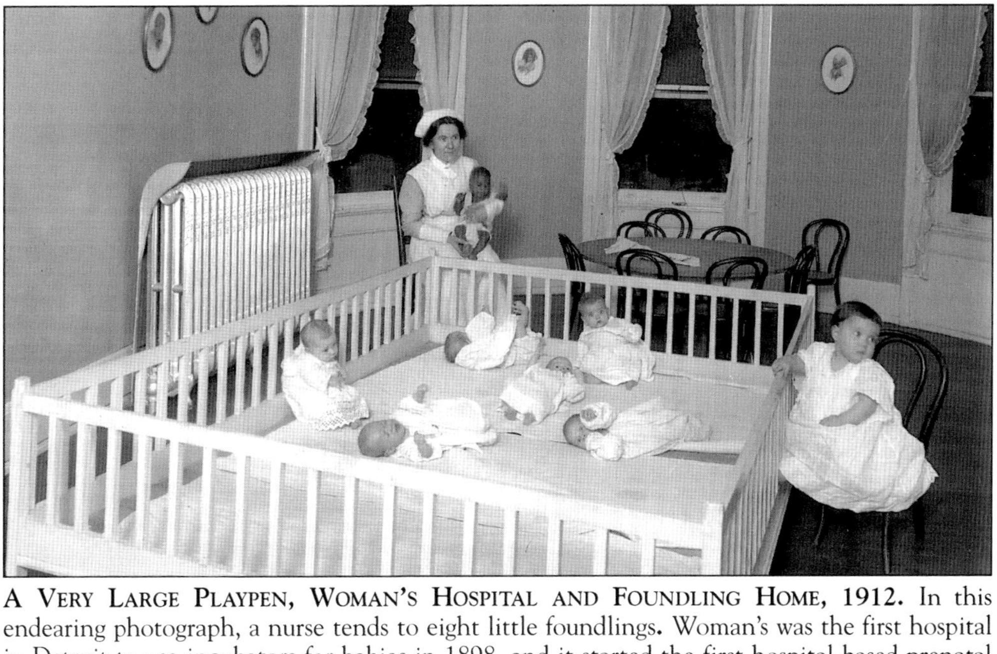

A VERY LARGE PLAYPEN, WOMAN'S HOSPITAL AND FOUNDLING HOME, 1912. In this endearing photograph, a nurse tends to eight little foundlings. Woman's was the first hospital in Detroit to use incubators for babies in 1898, and it started the first hospital-based prenatal clinics in 1915. (Courtesy Walter P. Reuther Library, Wayne State University.)

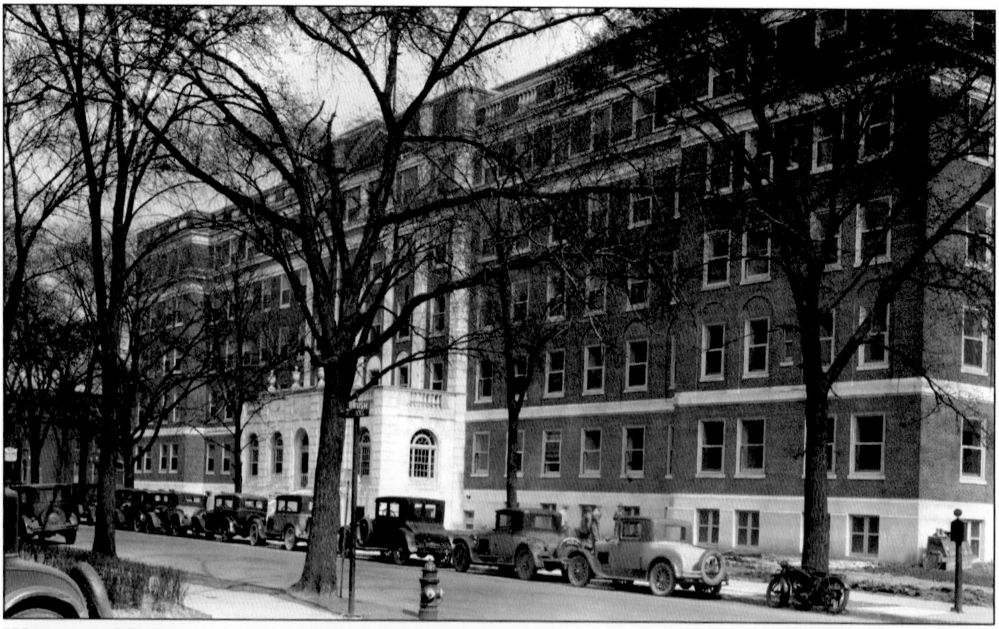

WOMAN'S HOSPITAL, 1929. The main entrance to the new hospital fronted on Hancock Street, and was surrounded by Forest, Beaubien, and Brush streets. During the Great Depression, out of economic necessity, the hospital started to admit men as patients and also offered medical and surgical services, but the primary role was always obstetrics and gynecology. (Courtesy Burton Historical Collection, Detroit Public Library.)

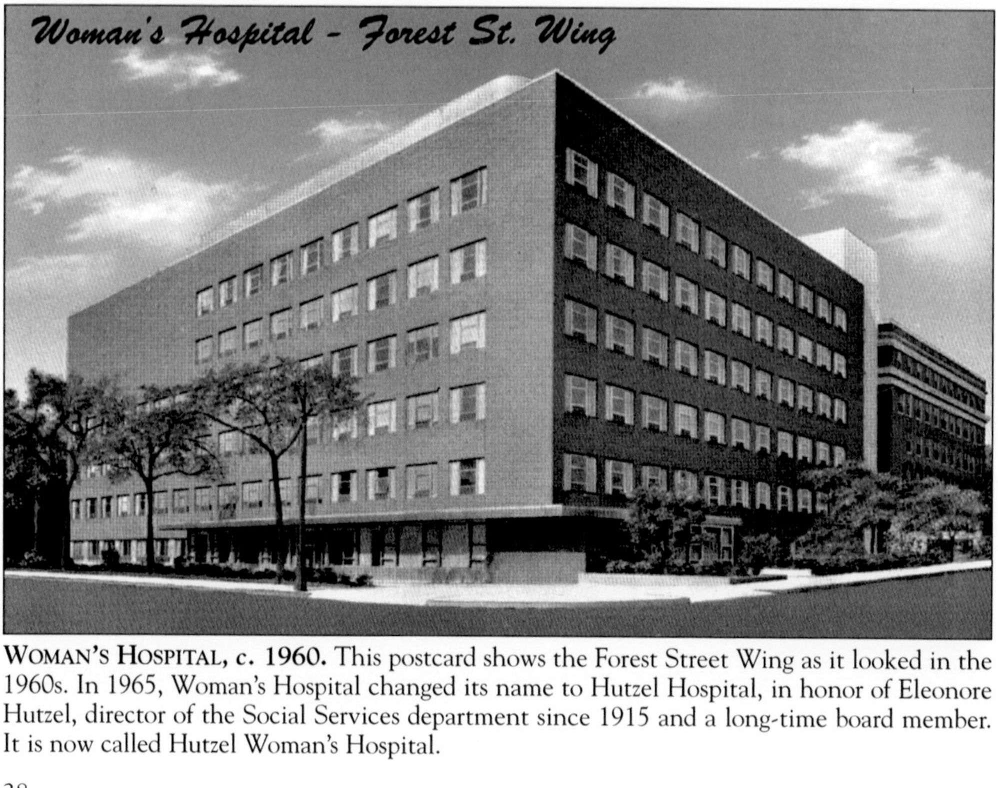

WOMAN'S HOSPITAL, c. 1960. This postcard shows the Forest Street Wing as it looked in the 1960s. In 1965, Woman's Hospital changed its name to Hutzel Hospital, in honor of Eleonore Hutzel, director of the Social Services department since 1915 and a long-time board member. It is now called Hutzel Woman's Hospital.

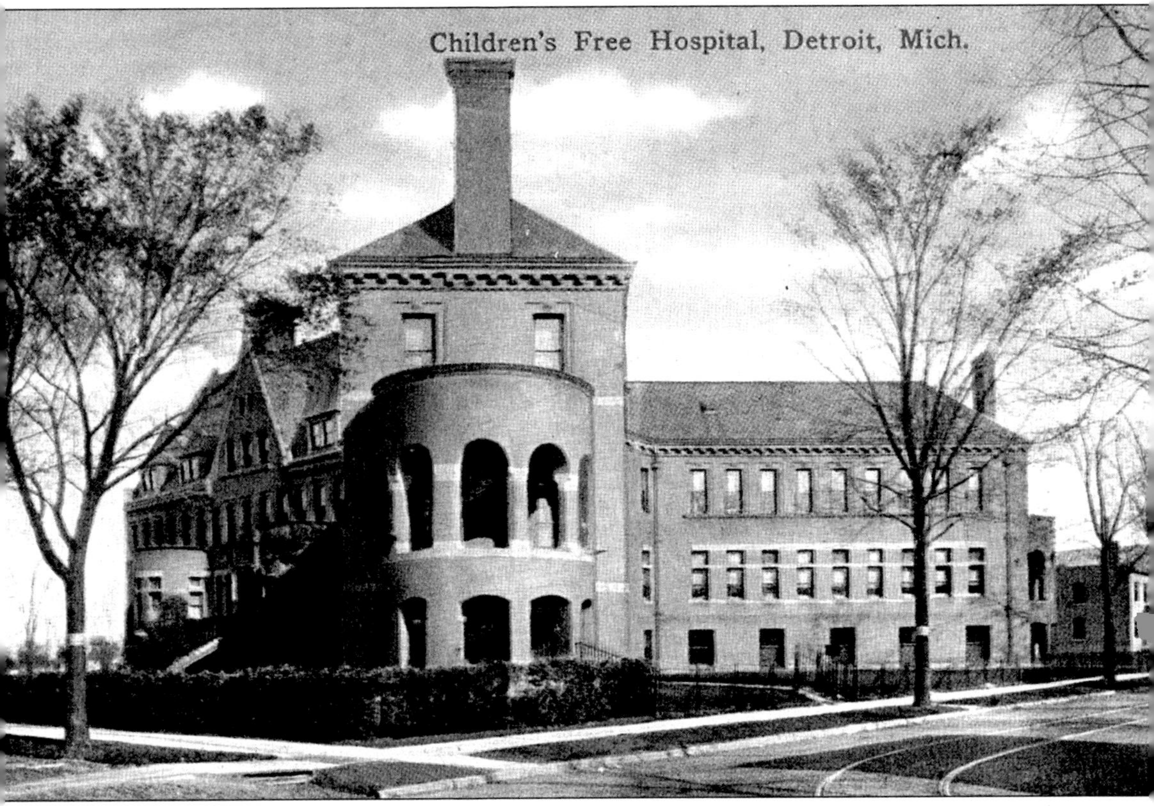

CHILDREN'S FREE HOSPITAL, c. 1909. It was Dr. Charles Devendorf, a Harper Hospital physician, who began a Children's Free Hospital on the ground floor of Harper Hospital to treat sick children regardless of race, religion, or ability to pay. It was Hiram Walker, a Canadian who is better known for his Canadian Club whisky business, who founded Children's Hospital in 1896 after he lost his 13-year-old daughter, Jennie Melissa. Walker bought the land and contributed $125,000 for the new hospital. This building stood at St. Antoine and Farnsworth Streets. (Courtesy Cheryl Strange-Laetsch.)

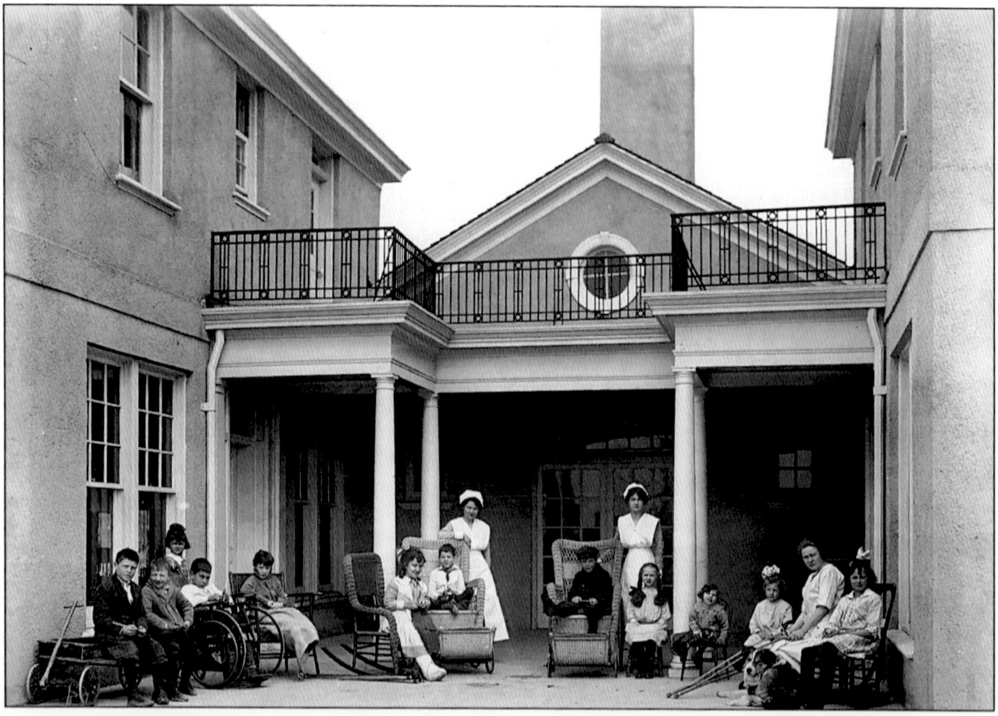

STAFF AND PATIENTS OF CHILDREN'S HOSPITAL, c. 1900. This wonderful glass negative of some nurses, their little patients, and their dog was probably taken outside of Children's Free Hospital. The expressions on the children's faces are both timeless and priceless. (Courtesy Burton Historical Collection, Detroit Public Library.)

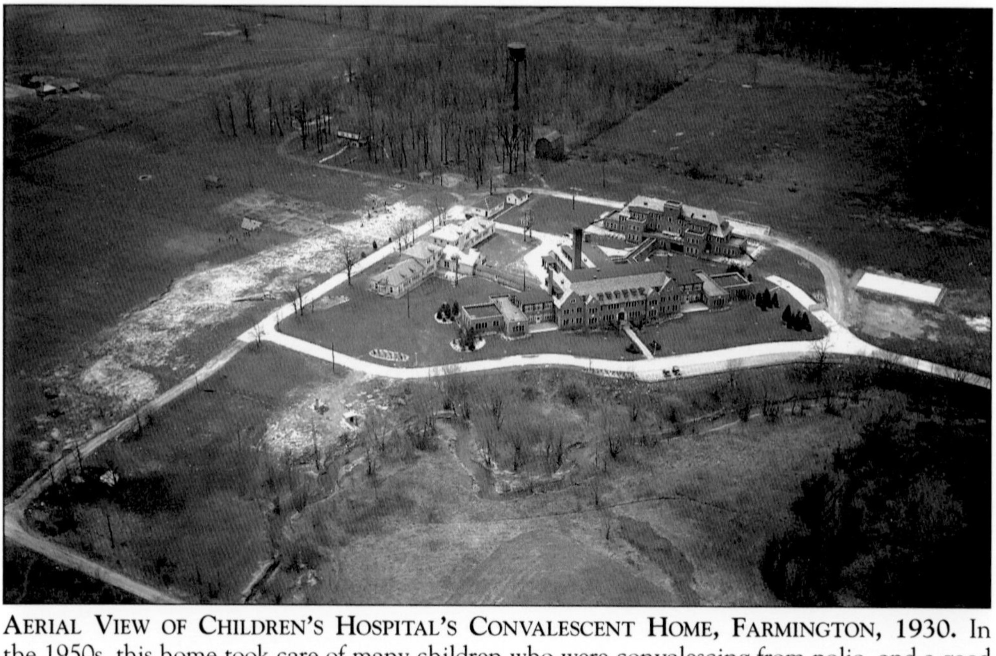

AERIAL VIEW OF CHILDREN'S HOSPITAL'S CONVALESCENT HOME, FARMINGTON, 1930. In the 1950s, this home took care of many children who were convalescing from polio, and a good number of them were teenagers. (Courtesy Walter P. Reuther Library, Wayne State University.)

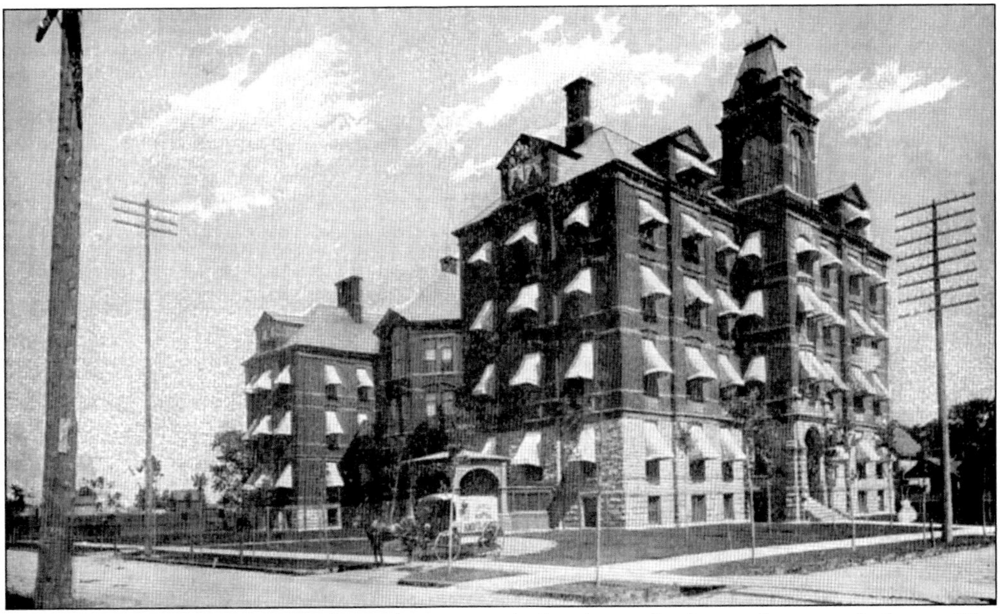

Grace Hospital, c. 1900. This color postcard also shows the horse-drawn ambulance. The great magician Harry Houdini died here in Room 401 on Halloween, 1926. Séances were held here annually on the anniversary of his death. This building was called Old Grace to differentiate it from the northwest branch which was built in 1942 and called New Grace. This building was used until 1978, and was torn down in 1980.

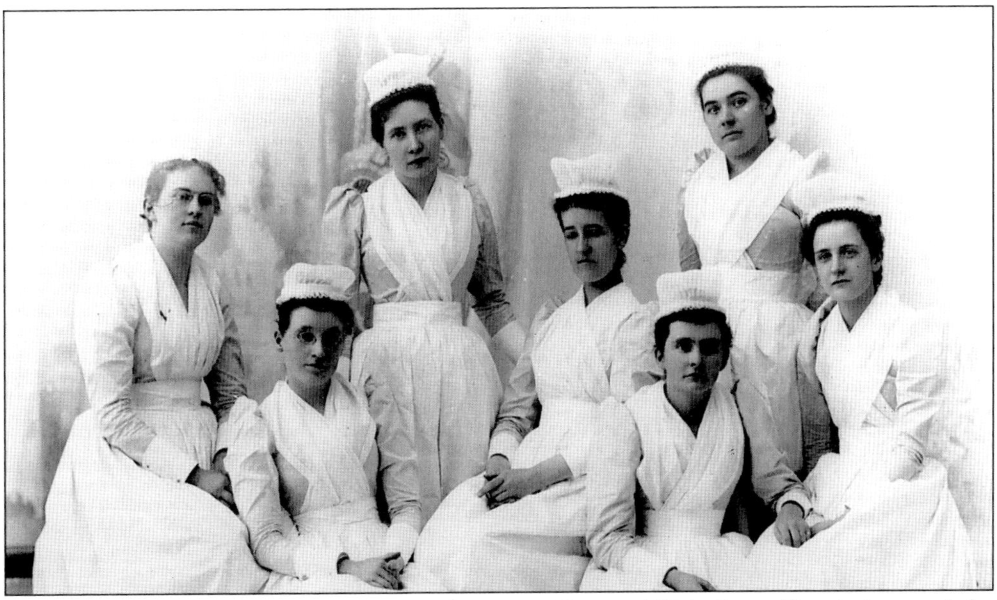

Grace Hospital School of Nursing, January Class, 1894. Grace Hospital opened the Grace Hospital Training School for Nurses in 1889, and the student nurses wore a distinctive pink uniform covered by a white bib apron. They were nicknamed "the pinkies." Shown here are, from left to right: (standing in rear) Ida C. White and Ellen May Tower; (front row) Martha Stark, Martha McVicar, E. Constance Fraser, Daisy Rutherford, and Lorain Smith. (Courtesy Walter P. Reuther Library, Wayne State University.)

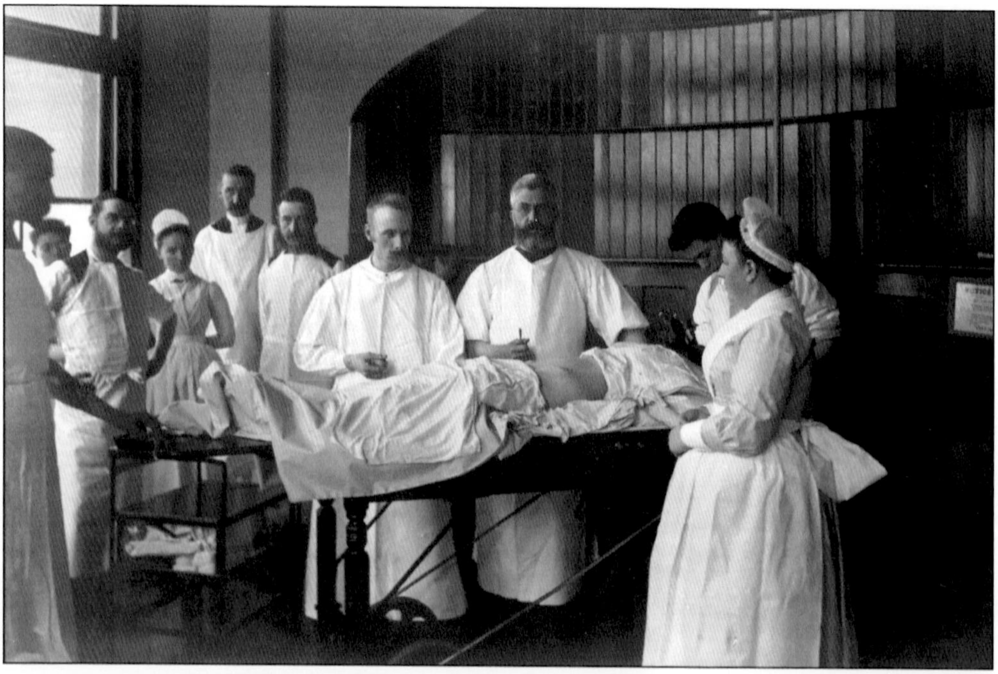

Operating Room, Grace Hospital, 1890. This hospital stood on the northeast corner of Willis Avenue and John R. Street on land donated by Amos Chafee in 1869 as a site for a homeopathic hospital. The hospital was named for the late daughter of one of the hospital's benefactors, Senator James McMillan. These photos show an operation in progress in the surgical amphitheatre. The wooden seating area behind the staff was for students and spectators. In one photo the patient is receiving a blood transfusion. (Courtesy Burton Historical Collection, Detroit Public Library.)

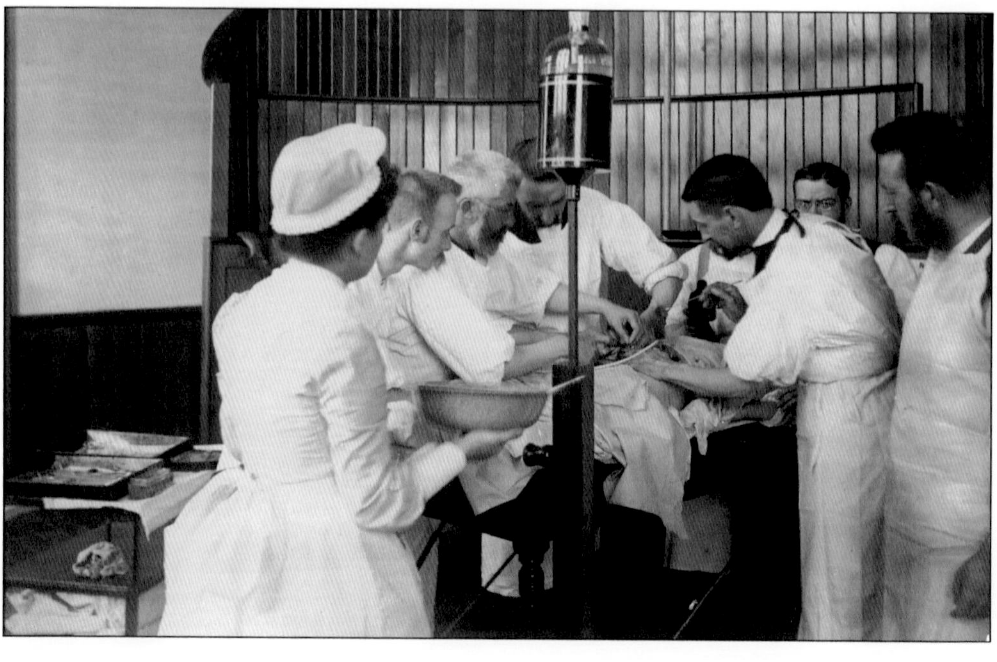

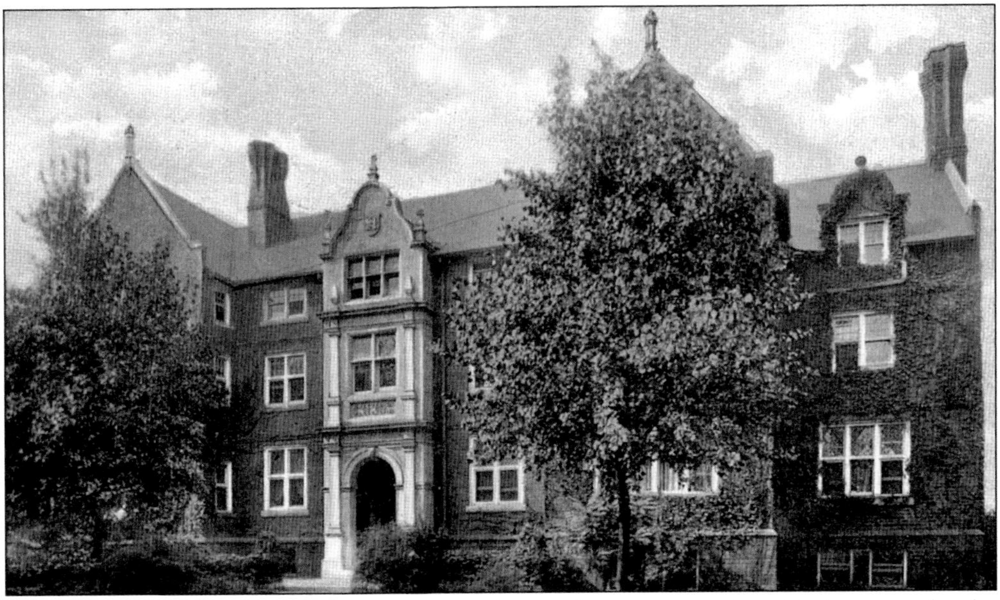

NURSES HOME, GRACE HOSPITAL, c. 1909. This color postcard printed in Germany by the Wolverine News Co. of Detroit, Michigan, shows the nurses' home which was replaced by a larger, more modern dwelling in 1930. The nursing school was closed in 1980. Grace Hospital graduated over 7,000 nurses from its diploma program in its 91 years of existence.

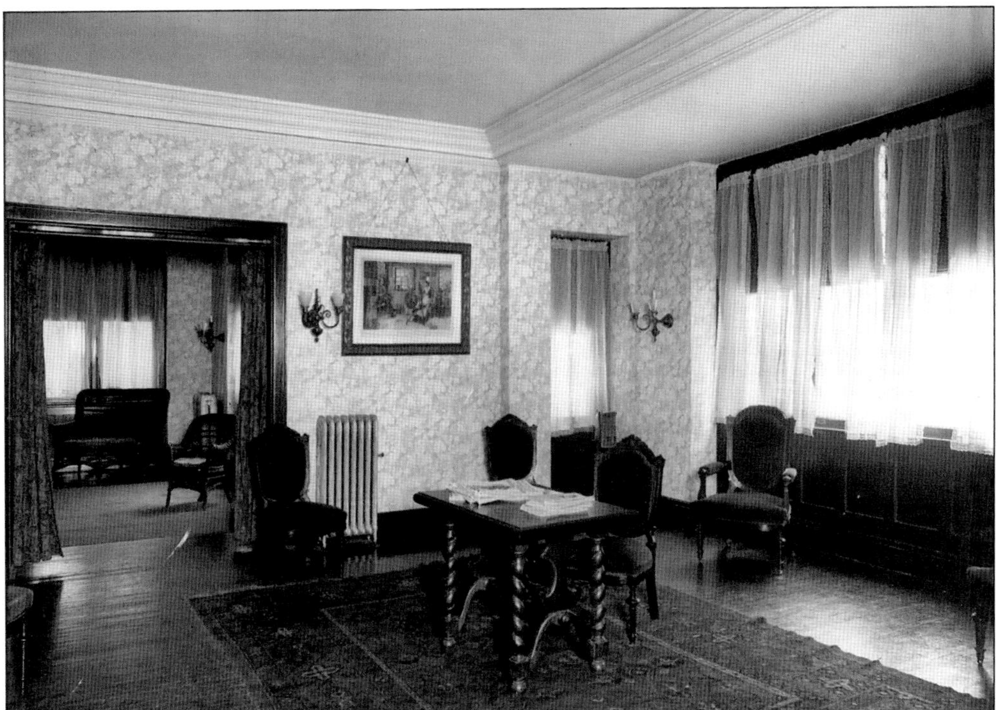

NURSES PARLOR, NURSES HOME, GRACE HOSPITAL, c. 1920. Most of the students and unmarried nurses lived in the nurses' home, and they entertained their guests or gentleman callers in this formal parlor. (Courtesy Walter P. Reuther Library, Wayne State University.)

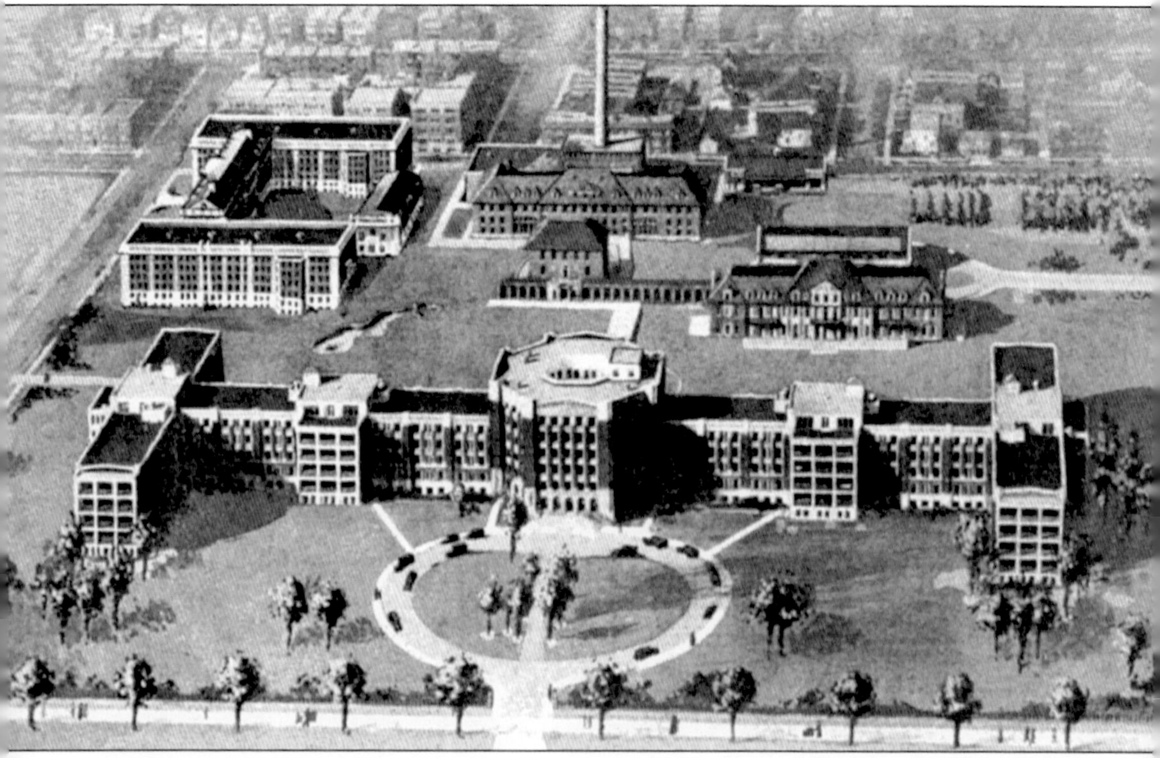

AERIAL VIEW OF HOSPITAL FOUNDED BY HENRY FORD, 1927. This large hospital complex, with nine buildings—including a power plant—first opened as a general hospital in 1915. It originally started as a subscription project in 1908, but was completed by Henry Ford when subscriptions failed to materialize. The hospital also ran a nursing school which operated for 71 years. The main hospital is still located at 2799 West Grand Boulevard and is now part of a major Michigan health care system.

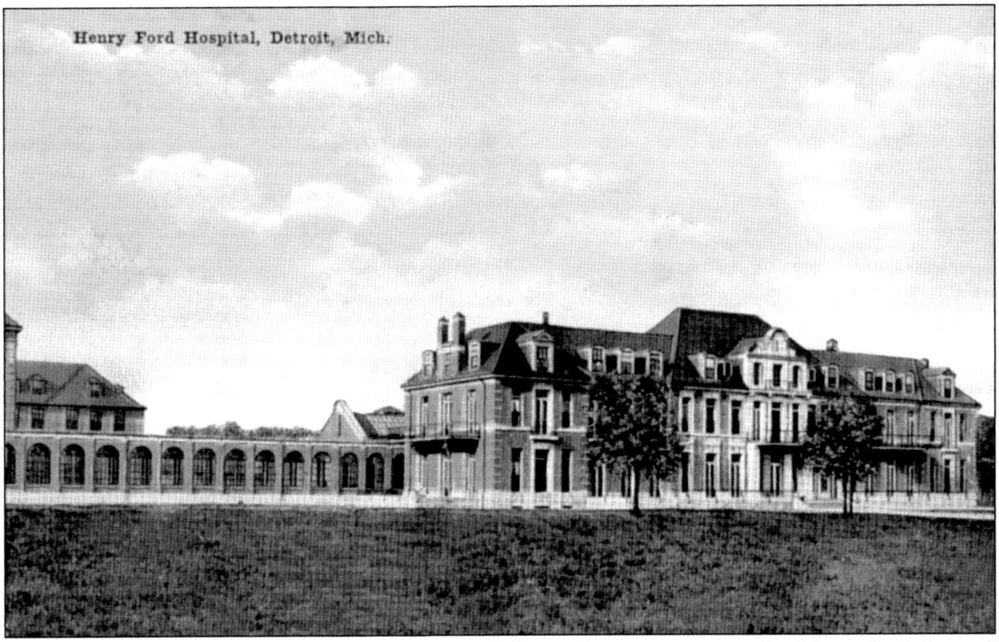

HENRY FORD HOSPITAL, c. 1915. This postcard shows the private patient building which housed only 48 patients. Henry Ford himself organized the medical staff, many of whom came from Johns Hopkins. Within two years, construction of a larger building began on this site, and during World War I the hospital was turned over to the government and was known as Base Hospital No. 36.

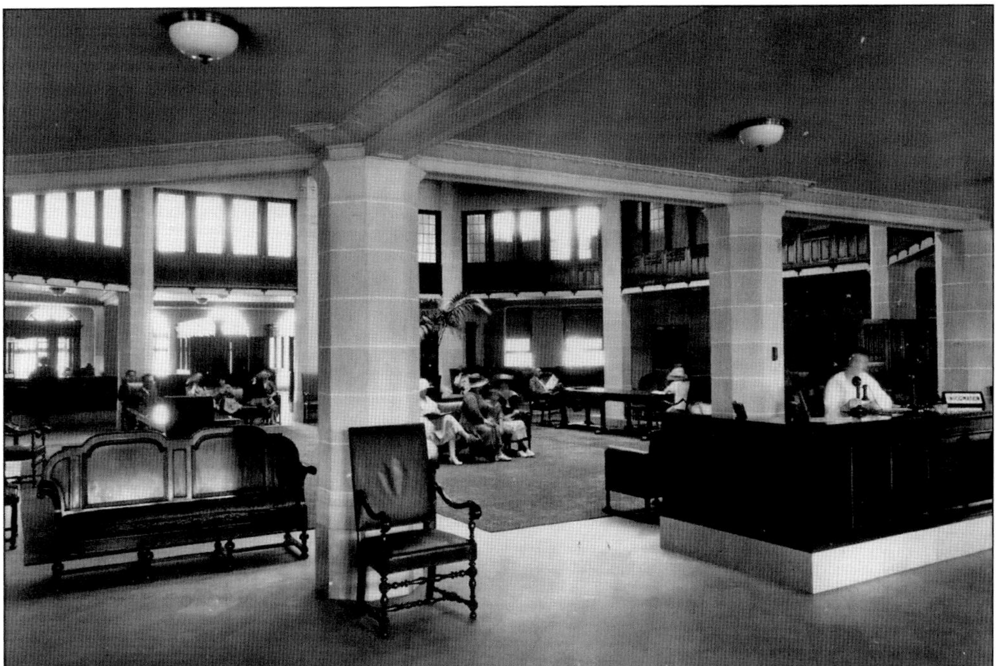

MAIN LOBBY OF HENRY FORD HOSPITAL, 1922. A gentleman is leisurely reading his newspaper in what looks like the lobby of a fine hotel. (Courtesy Burton Historical Collection, Detroit Public Library.)

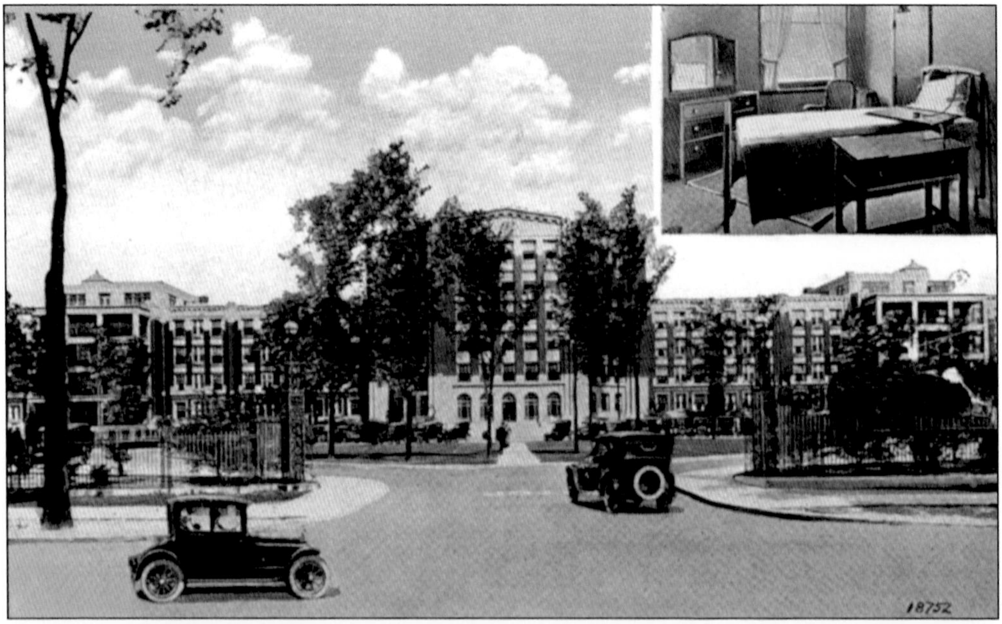

WEST GRAND BOULEVARD ENTRANCE TO HENRY FORD HOSPITAL, 1926. After World War I, the 50,000 square foot building was completed and provided 500 hospital beds to Detroit, which was then a rapidly growing city. The postcard insert shows a patient room typical of the time.

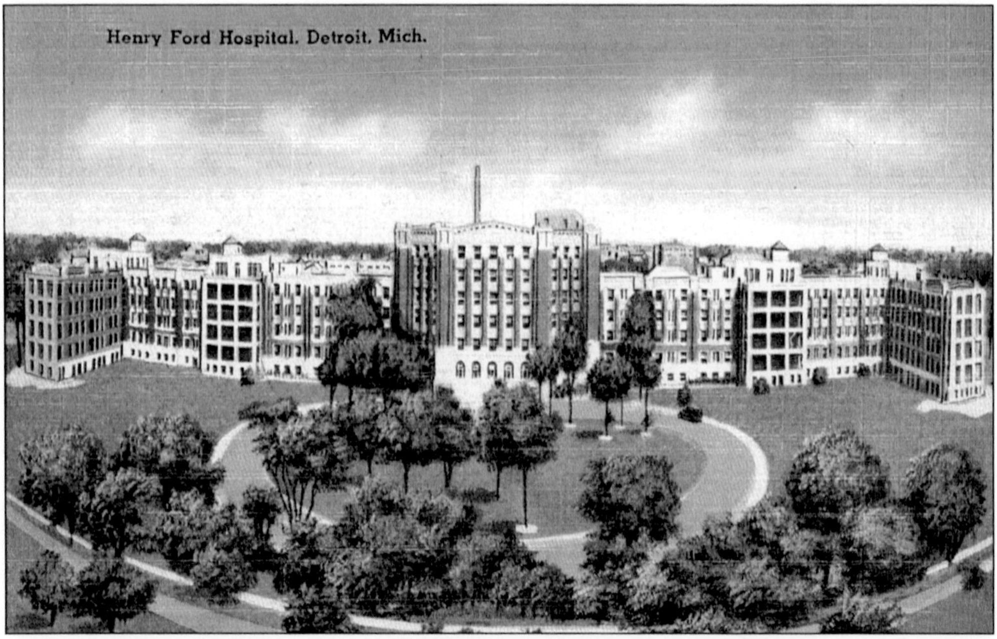

ANOTHER VIEW OF HENRY FORD HOSPITAL, c. 1930. Henry Ford Hospital was a popular subject for postcards, and this view shows the main hospital building. Henry Ford intended this hospital to be one of the largest and best-equipped hospitals in the U.S.

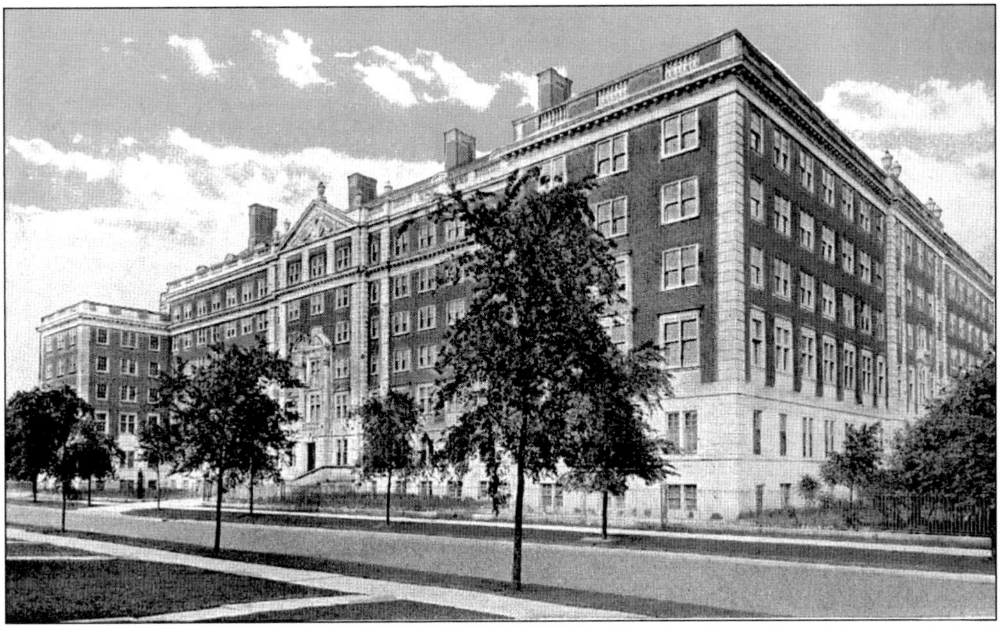

Clara Ford Nurses' Home, 1925. This nurses' home for the Henry Ford Hospital School of Nursing and Hygiene was added to the hospital in 1925, and provided very beautiful and spacious quarters to the 91 nurses who lived there. It had 300 rooms, and it even had a gymnasium and swimming pool. The building is now called the Clara Ford Pavilion and is used for medical and business offices.

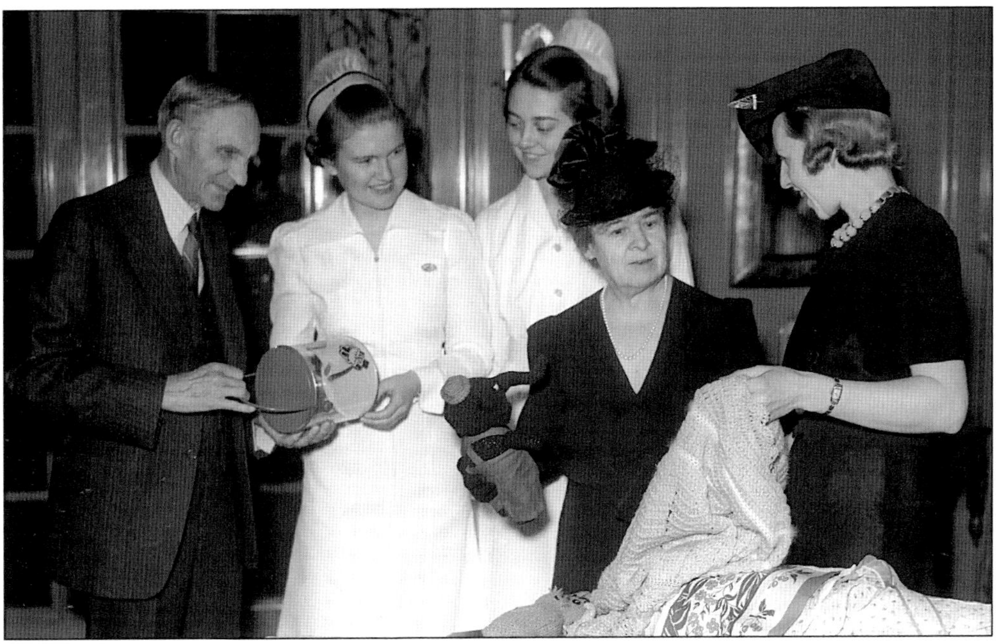

Henry and Clara Ford at the Clara Ford Nurses' Home, 1939. The Fords are admiring some craft items in one of the parlors of the nurses' home named for Mrs. Ford, while two Henry Ford graduate nurses and an unidentified woman assist. Ford grads were recognized by their unique caps. (Courtesy Walter P. Reuther Library, Wayne State University.)

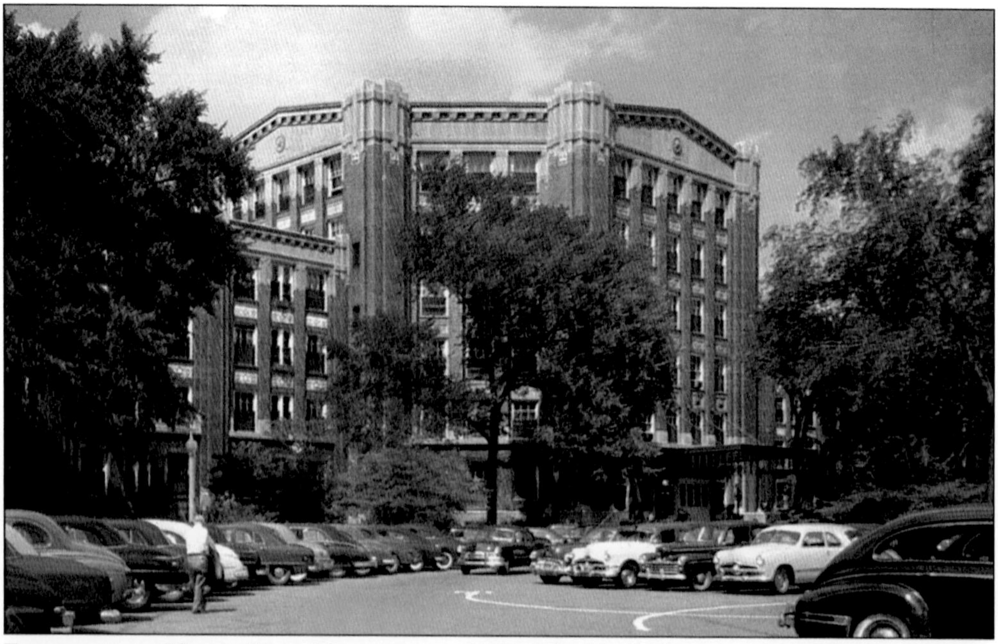

ENTRANCE TO HENRY FORD HOSPITAL, c. 1950. The hospital grew as Detroit grew, and this color postcard shows how it looked in the mid-20th century.

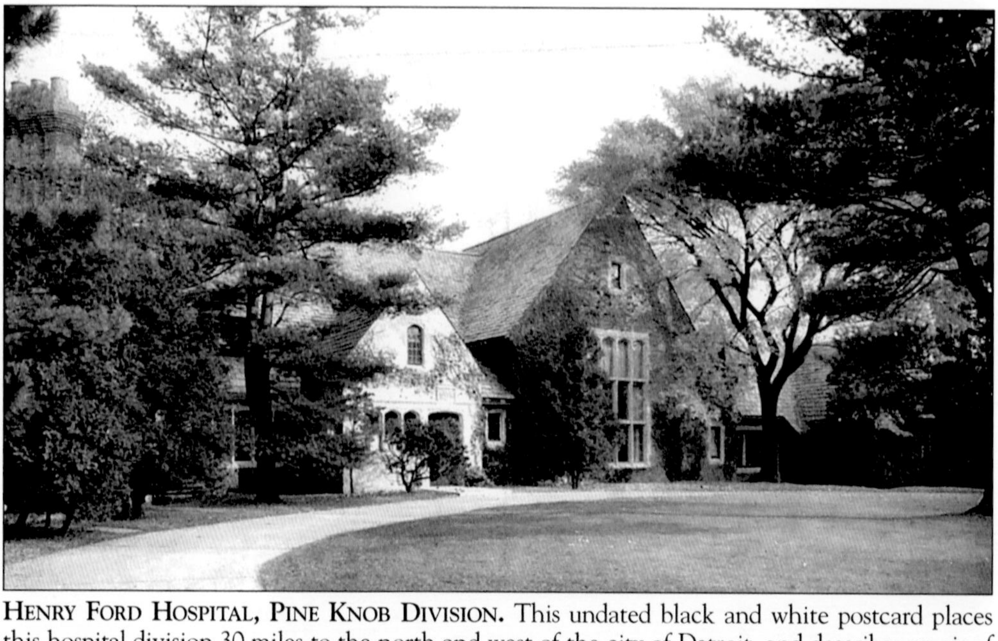

HENRY FORD HOSPITAL, PINE KNOB DIVISION. This undated black and white postcard places this hospital division 30 miles to the north and west of the city of Detroit, and describes an air of quiet restfulness. It was originally the home of Col. and Mrs. Sidney Waldon, and it was used for orthopedic, psychiatric, pediatric, and postoperative patients. (Courtesy Cheryl Strange-Laetsch.)

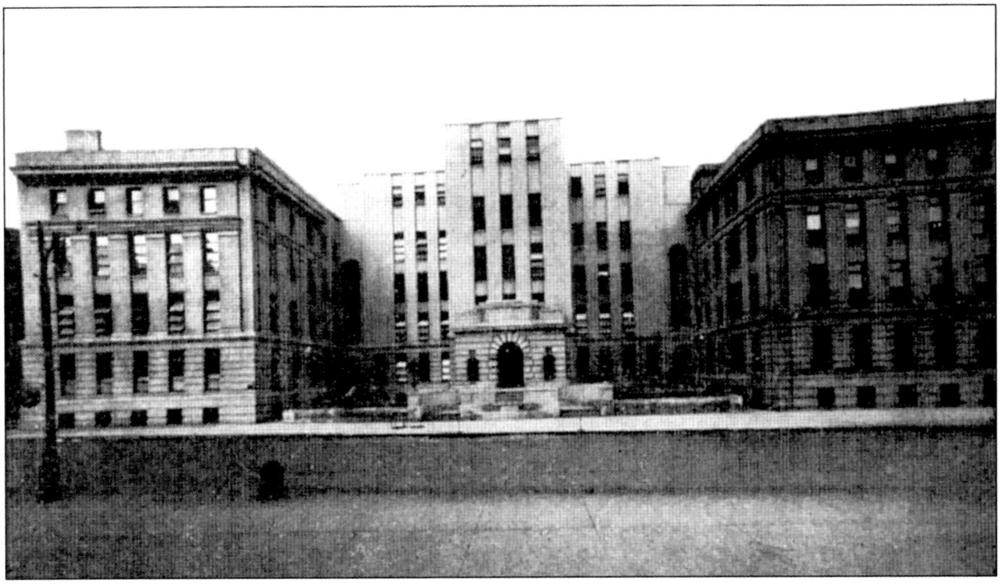

DETROIT RECEIVING HOSPITAL, c. 1927. Detroit Receiving Hospital was run by the Public Welfare Commission of the City of Detroit, and it was located at St. Antoine at Macomb and Clinton Streets. It had 593 beds and was an emergency and psychiatric hospital. Thomas K. Gruber, M.D., was the superintendent here before he became the superintendent at Eloise.

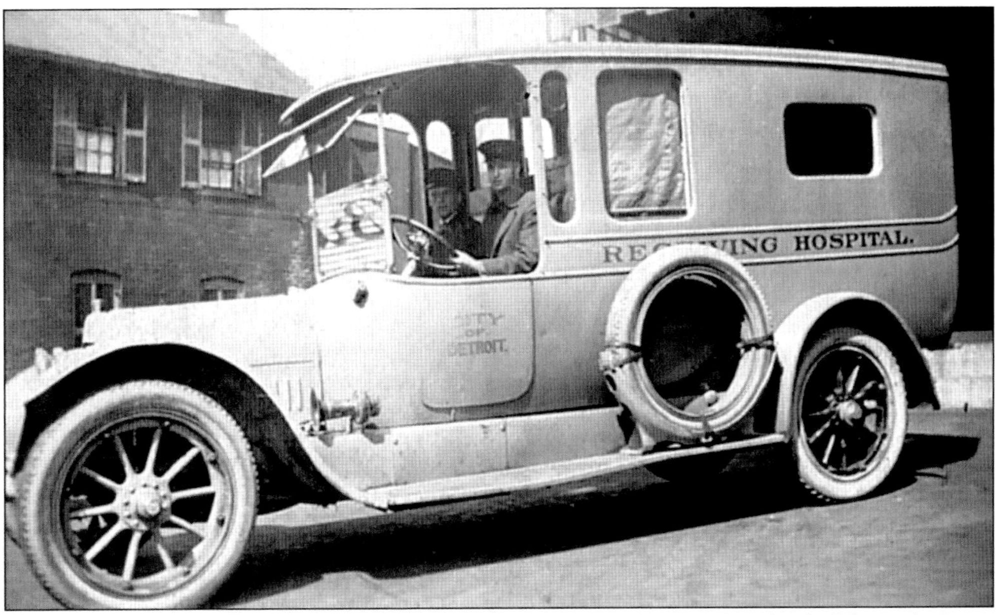

RECEIVING HOSPITAL AMBULANCE, 1920S. Baden Hudson is behind the wheel of this ambulance which apparently was later used at Eloise Hospital. (Courtesy Westland Historical Museum.)

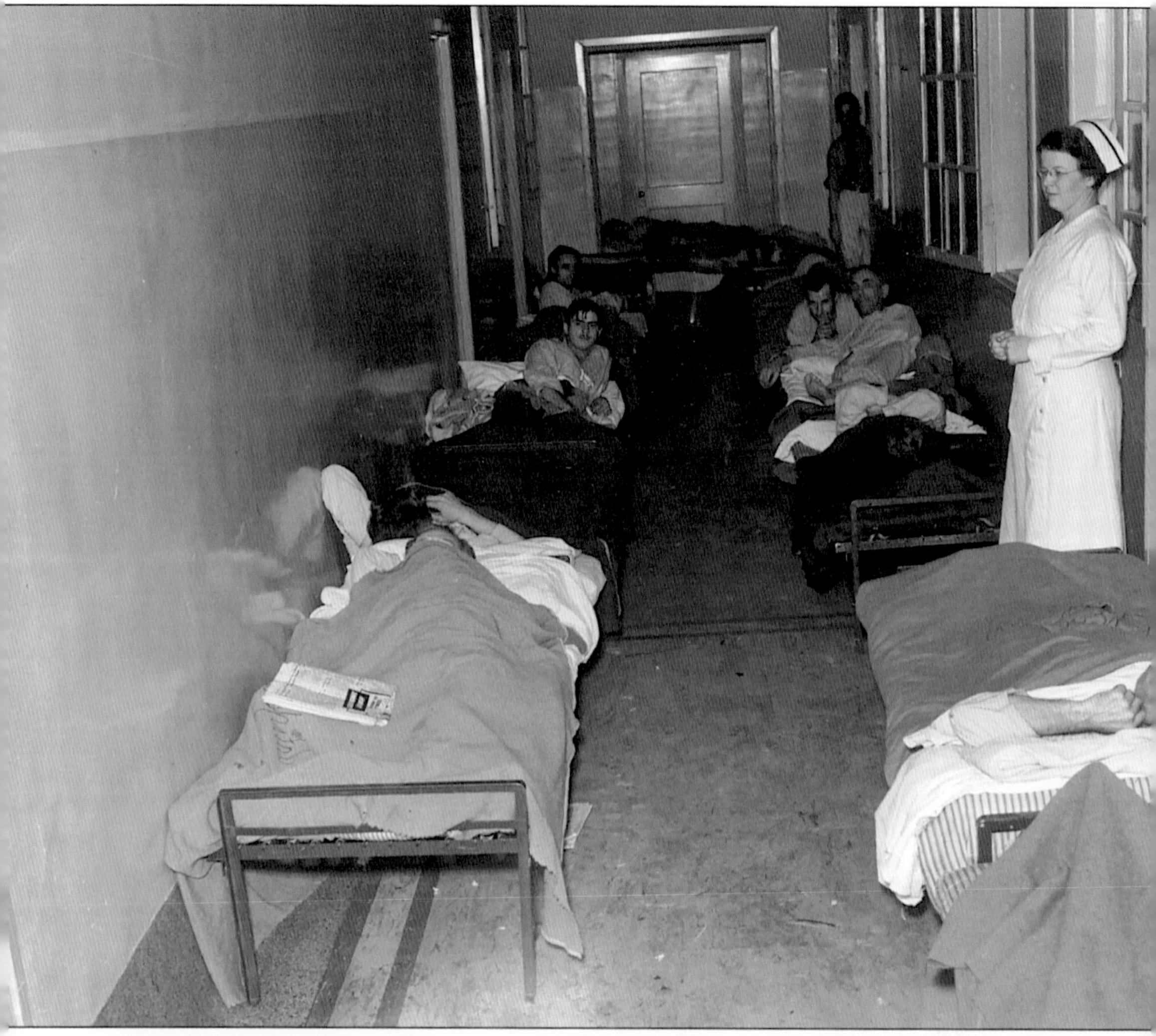

CROWDED CONDITIONS IN PSYCHOPATHIC WARD, 1937. A nurse observes male psychiatric patients who are resting on cots in a hallway at Detroit Receiving Hospital. Overcrowding was a serious problem in area psychiatric hospitals at the time as all the state asylums were full. (Courtesy Walter P. Reuther Library, Wayne State University.)

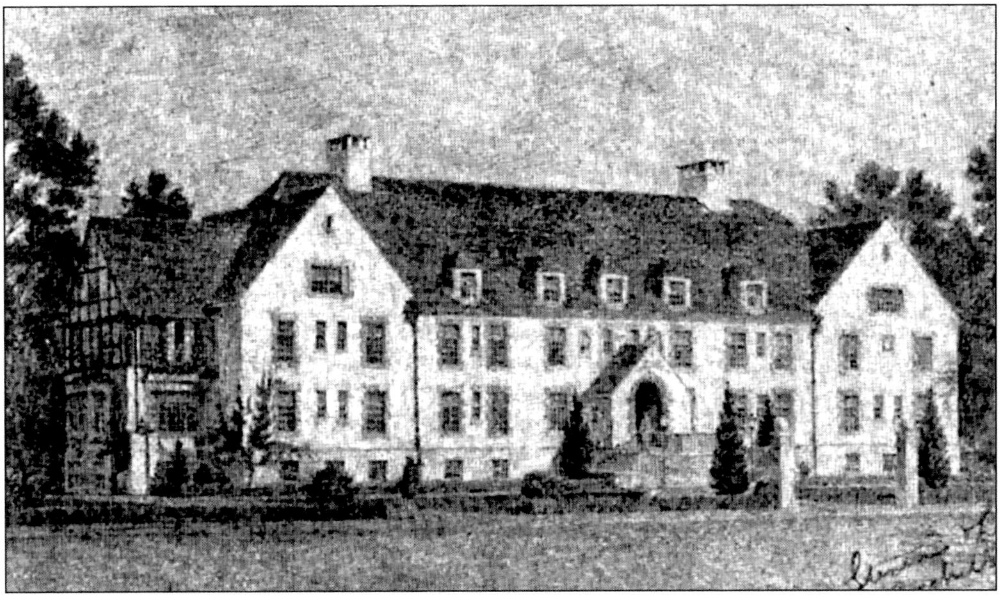

COTTAGE HOSPITAL, GROSSE POINTE, 1927. This 21-bed small community hospital was located at 54 Oak Street in Grosse Pointe. Mrs. J.P. Bernard, R.N., was the superintendent. It was opened in an eight-room house during the flu epidemic of 1917, and was expanded into a new 50-bed hospital in 1928.

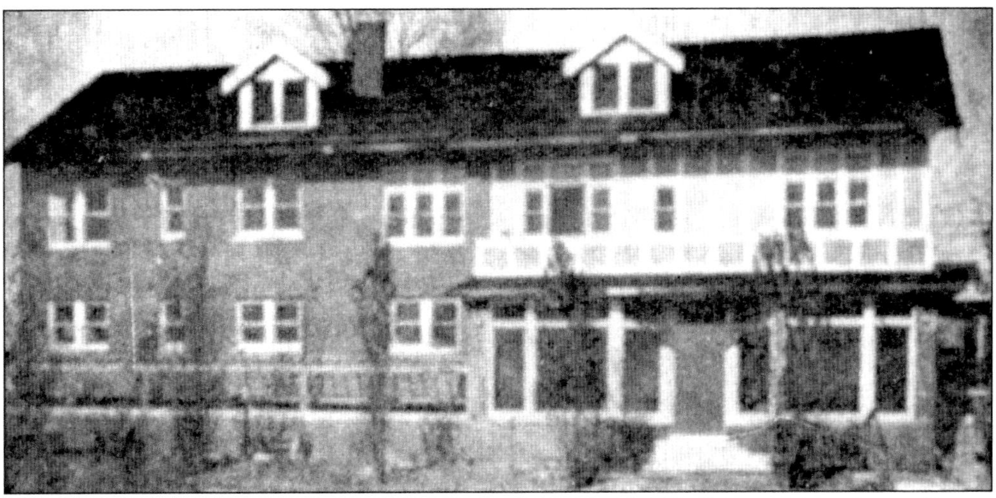

GROSSE POINTE HOSPITAL, 1927. This was another small 22-bed hospital in Grosse Pointe which was used for obstetrics and emergency.

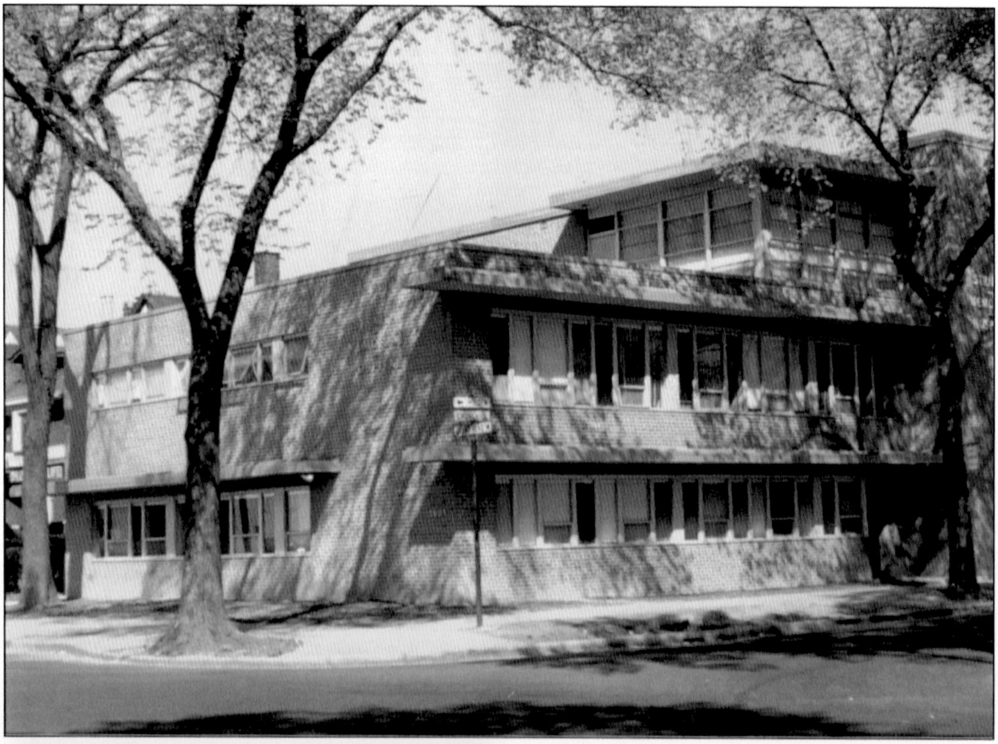

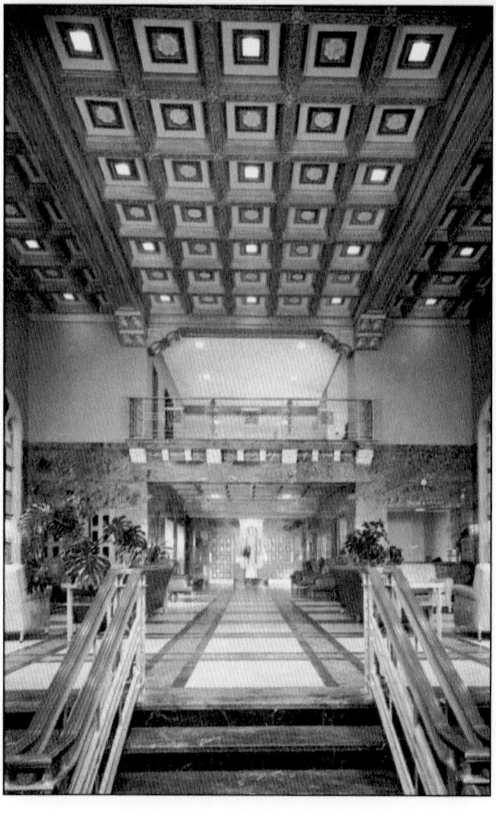

STRAITH MEMORIAL HOSPITAL, 1954. This hospital was located on Grand Boulevard and Churchill in Detroit. It opened in 1954 and specialized in the field of cosmetic and plastic surgery. It was founded by Claire Straith, M.D., D.D.S., and his son Richard Straith, M.D. The current hospital is located on Lahser Road in Southfield and was renamed the Straith Hospital for Special Surgery. (Courtesy Janet Husband.)

MAIN LOBBY OF ST. JOHN'S HOSPITAL. This color postcard shows the entrance into the main lobby of the hospital as it looked when it had recently opened.

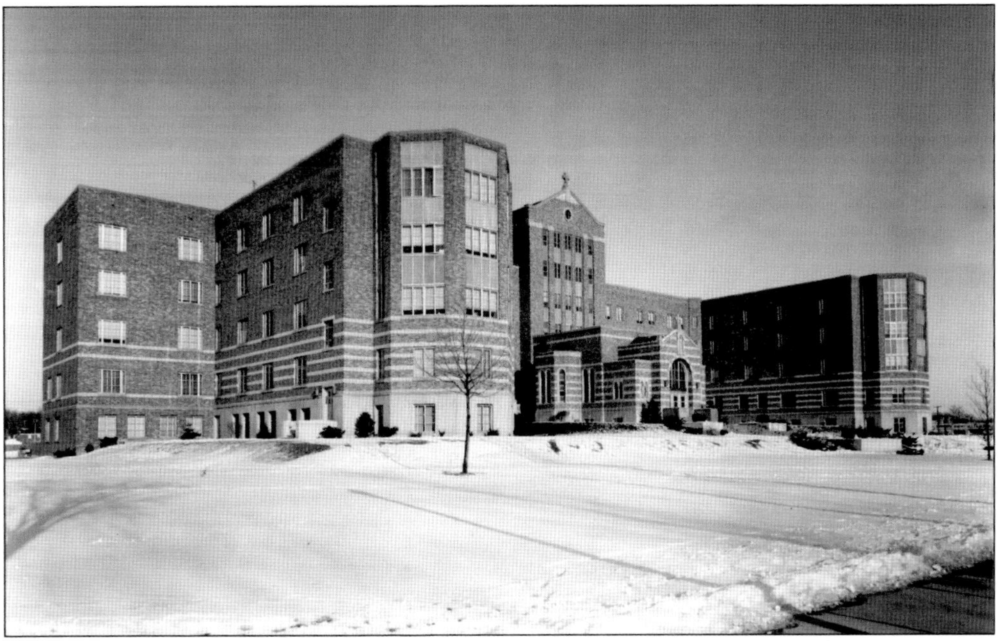

ST. JOHN'S HOSPITAL, 1956. St. John's was founded in 1952 by the Sisters of St. Joseph of Nazareth, Michigan. The 607-bed hospital at 22101 Moross on the east side of Detroit is part of the large St. John Health System, a network of eight hospitals in metro Detroit, which includes Providence as well as the former Detroit Memorial (St. Mary's), Alexander Blain, Jennings, and Detroit Osteopathic. (Courtesy Burton Historical Collection, Detroit Public Library.)

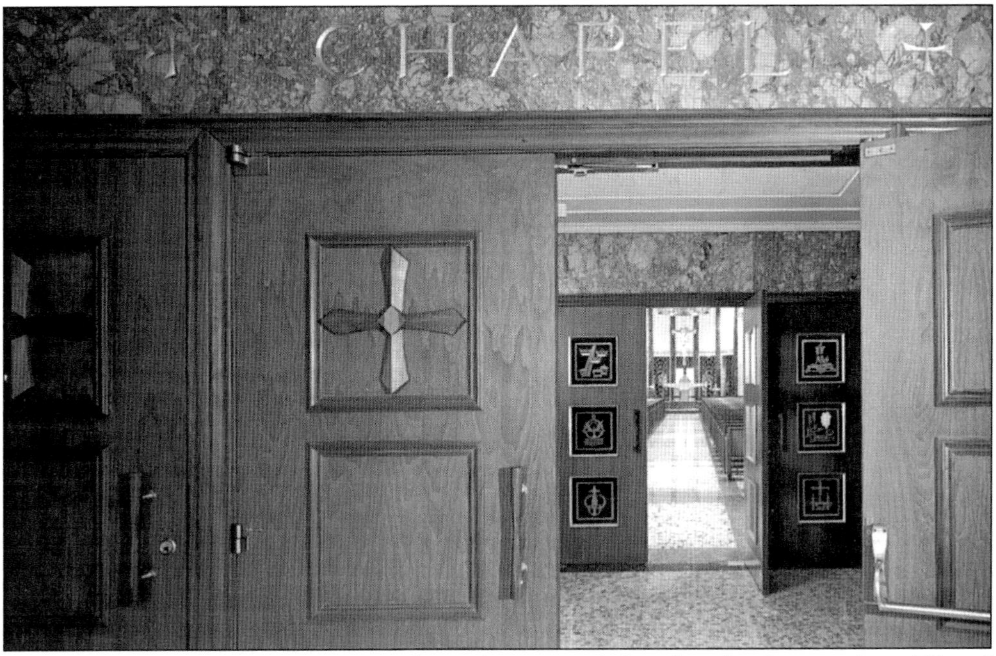

CHAPEL, ST. JOHN'S HOSPITAL. Another color postcard describes the doors to Saint Edward Chapel that are of carved wood from Ortisei, Italy. The ground glass symbolic panels in the doors are original designs from Munich, Germany.

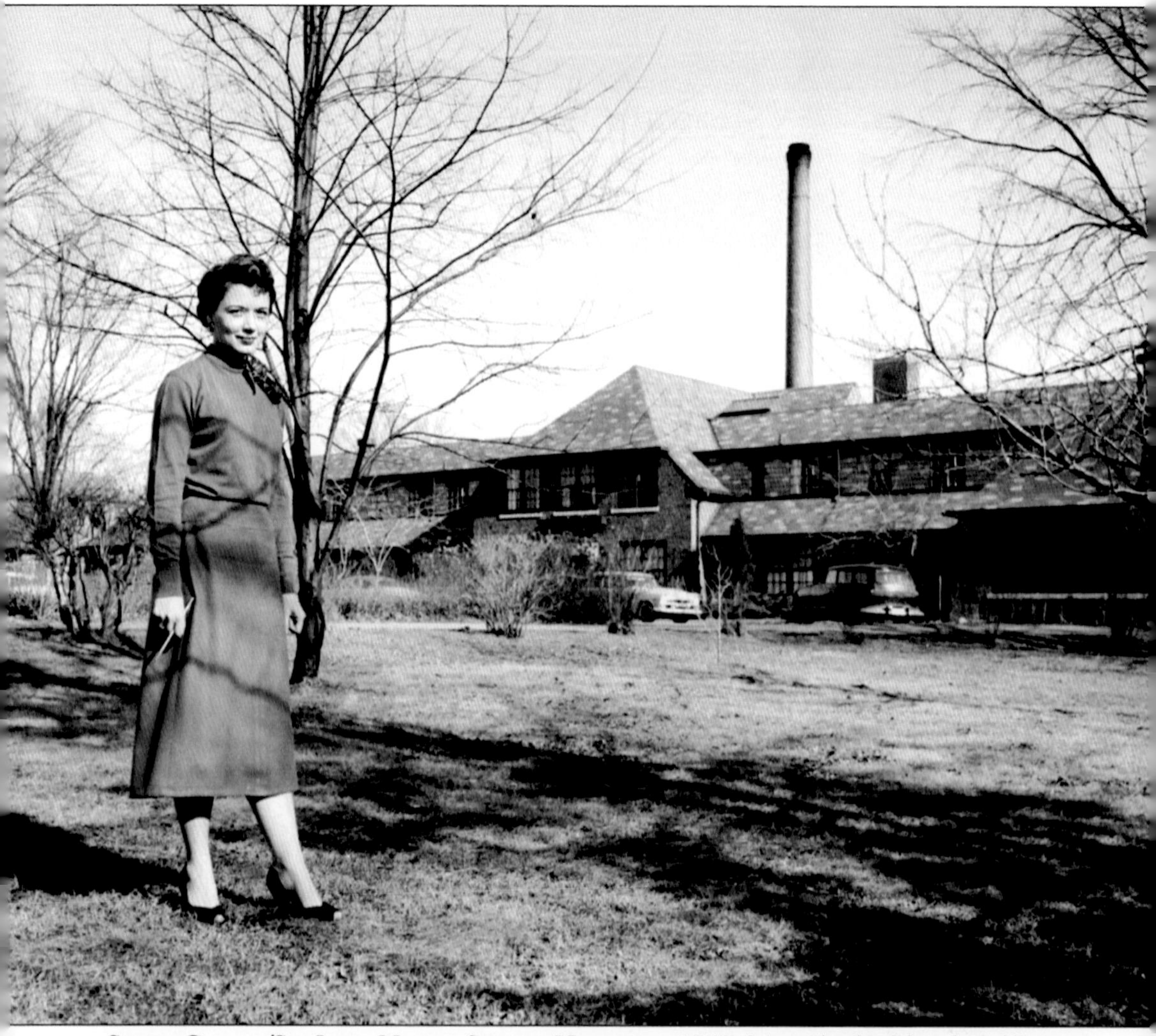

SIGMA GAMMA/ST. JOHN NORTH SHORES HOSPITAL, 1957. Mrs. Charles Rhoades of Detroit, a secretary at the hospital, is pictured standing in front of what was then the Sigma Gamma Hospital. It was designed by noted architect Albert Kahn. This hospital was built in 1925, and operated by members of the Sigma Gamma Sorority of Grosse Pointe. It was officially called the Memorial Orthopedic Hospital, and was a branch of the Detroit Orthopedic Hospital. It was used to treat young polio patients. Most of the employees of the hospital lived on the second floor. It closed in 1957 when there was a sharp decline in polio cases because of the Salk vaccine. Since that time, it has been used as a series of community hospitals, and is now St. John North Shores Hospital. (Courtesy Mount Clemens Public Library.)

Two

SANITARIUMS AND ASYLUMS

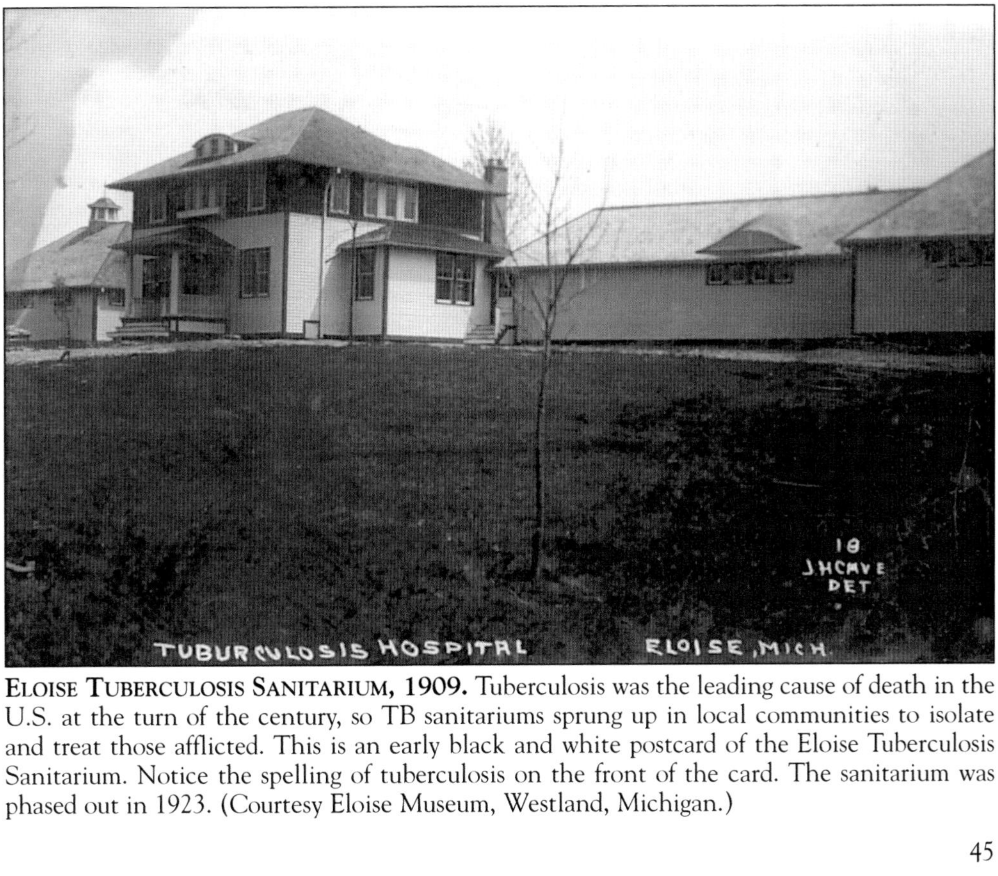

ELOISE TUBERCULOSIS SANITARIUM, 1909. Tuberculosis was the leading cause of death in the U.S. at the turn of the century, so TB sanitariums sprung up in local communities to isolate and treat those afflicted. This is an early black and white postcard of the Eloise Tuberculosis Sanitarium. Notice the spelling of tuberculosis on the front of the card. The sanitarium was phased out in 1923. (Courtesy Eloise Museum, Westland, Michigan.)

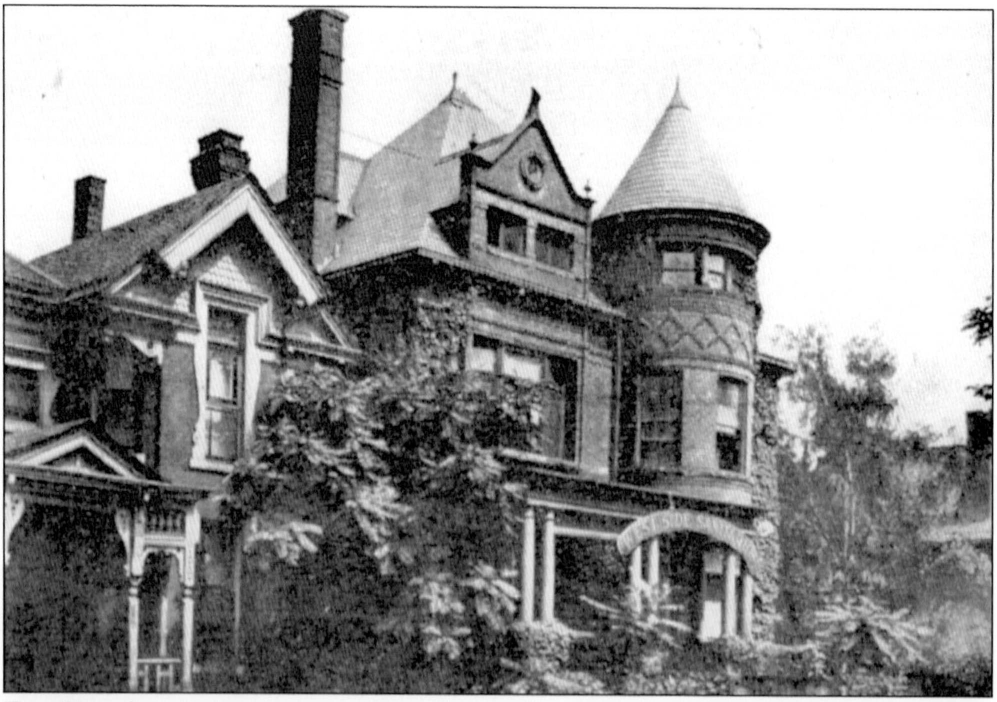

The West Side Sanitarium, c. 1927. This small sanitarium was located at 3840 Fort Street, and was an 18-bed private mental hospital which specialized in the treatment of alcoholic, drug, and mental patients. The doctor in charge in 1927 was J.R. Rupp, M.D.

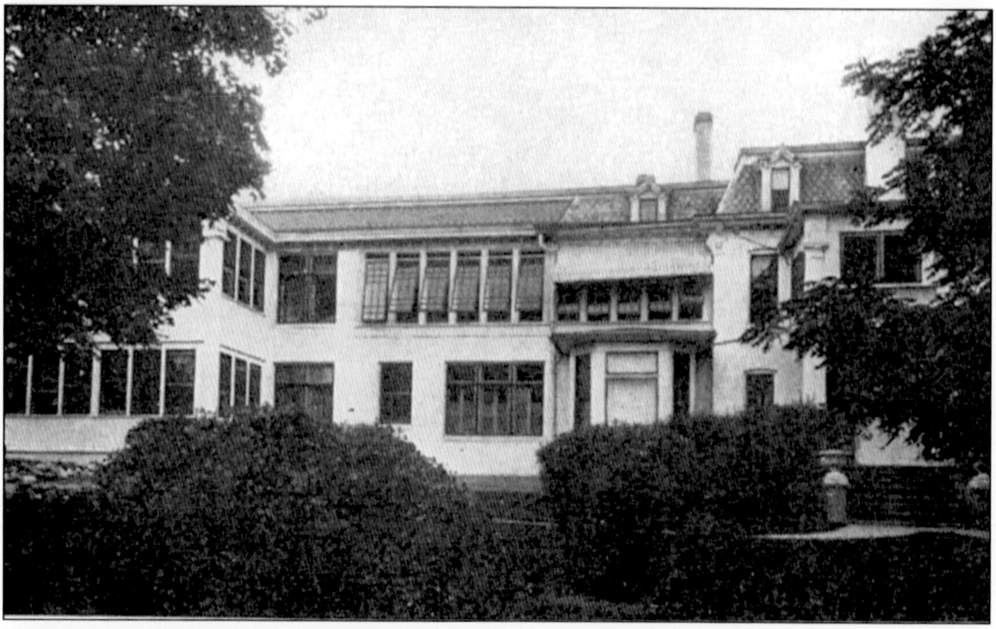

East Lawn Sanitarium, c. 1927. This 65-bed tuberculosis sanitarium was located in Northville, Michigan. To get there in 1927, Detroit residents had to take the Northville bus, leaving the Campus Martius in front of the Shubert Theater. The bus schedule was available at the Information Desk in the Book-Cadillac Hotel.

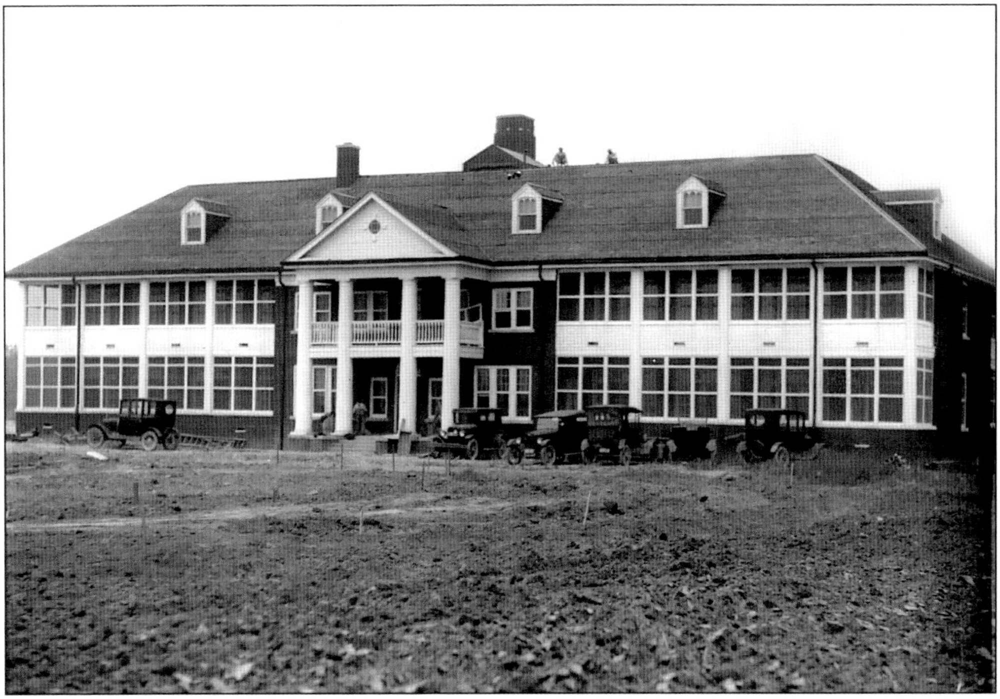

FRANK B. LELAND FARM AT YPSILANTI, c. 1926. Workers are putting the finishing touches on this sanitarium in Ypsilanti which opened in 1926 and was an annex of the Detroit Tuberculosis Sanitarium. About 100 incipient and aftercare cases were treated here. Fresh air and sunshine were believed to be beneficial to patients with tuberculosis. (Courtesy Walter P. Reuther Library, Wayne State University.)

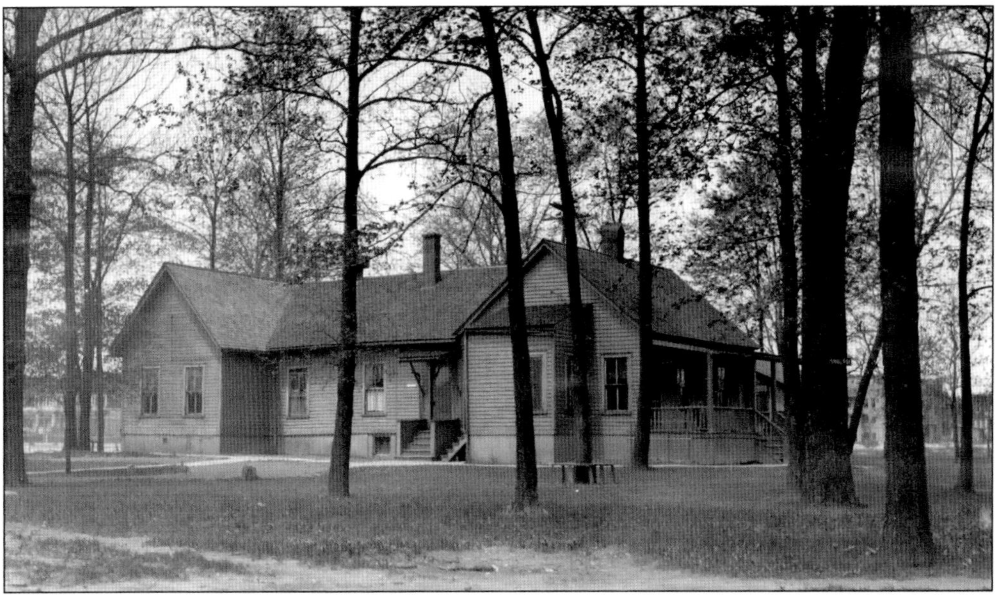

SMALLPOX BUILDING, HERMAN KIEFER HOSPITAL. This frame building was used to isolate patients with smallpox, which is highly contagious, and was part of the Kiefer complex on the then-wooded grounds of the hospital. (Courtesy Burton Historical Collection, Detroit Public Library.)

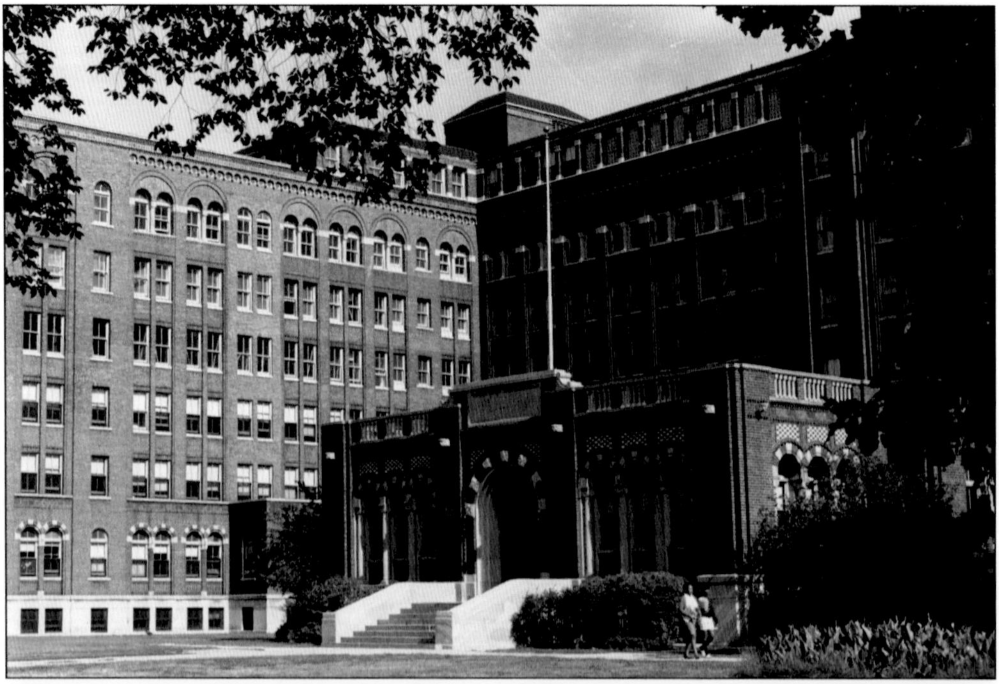

Herman Kiefer Hospital, 1920s. Herman Kiefer was an eminent physician and author. The hospital on Hamilton Boulevard, which was named for him and run by the Detroit Health Department, had a tuberculosis division which was established in 1911. The hospital also cared for patients with polio and other communicable diseases. The complex included an obstetrical hospital, a nurses' residence, and several other buildings. (Courtesy Burton Historical Collection, Detroit Public Library.)

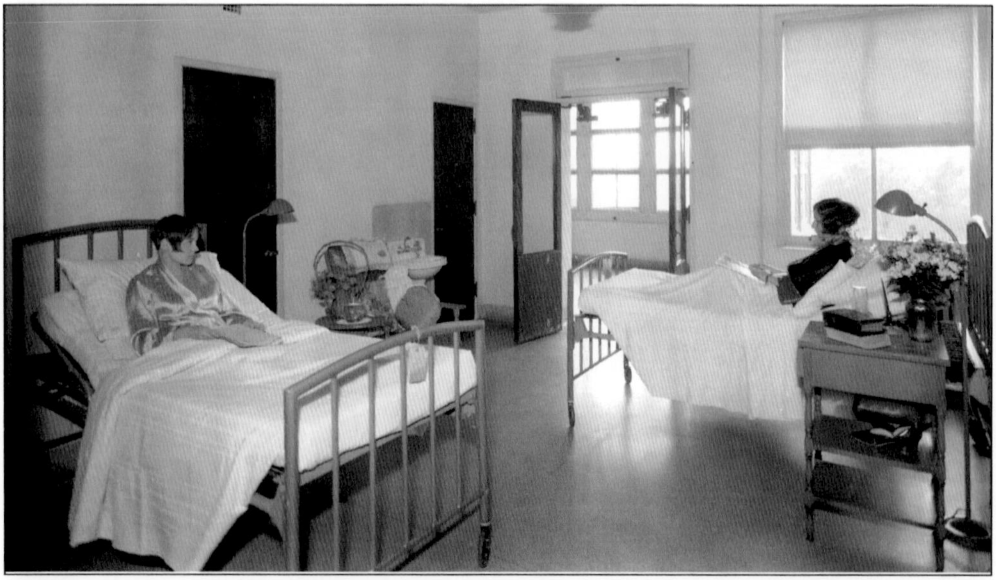

Patient Room, Herman Kiefer Hospital, 1920s. These ladies sporting the fashionable bob haircuts of the 1920s are resting in a semi-private room in the main hospital building. (Courtesy Burton Historical Collection, Detroit Public Library.)

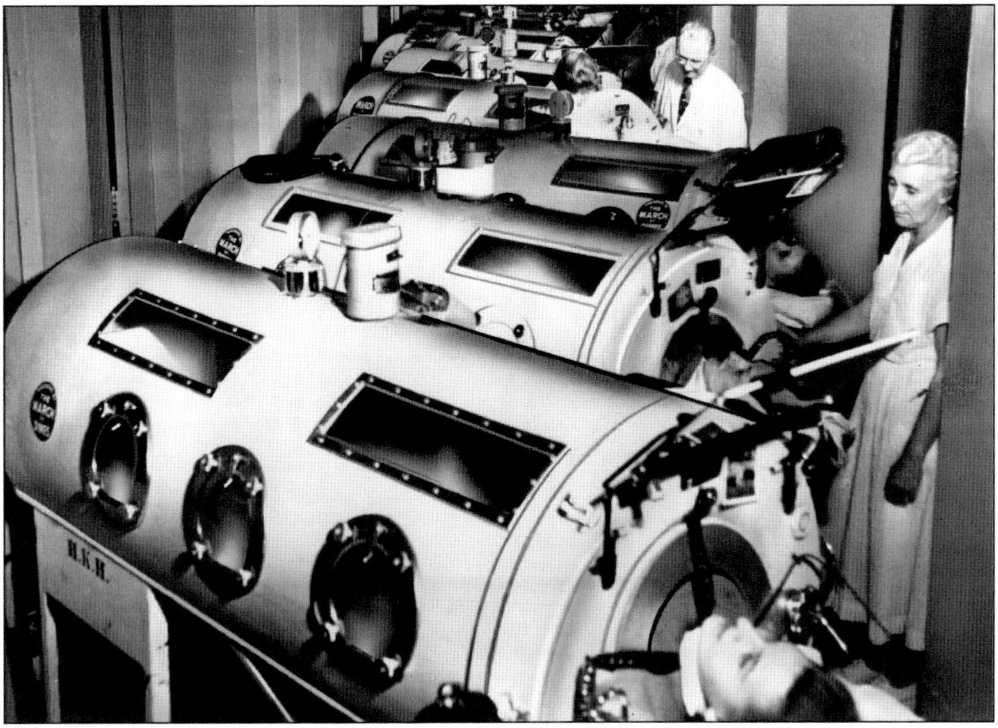

VICTIMS OF THE POLIO EPIDEMIC, 1950S. Polio is almost extinct now, but it was a major illness in the 1950s, and patients were placed in iron lungs to help them breathe. Here a doctor and nurse attend to a row of patients in iron lungs at Herman Kiefer Hospital. (Courtesy Burton Historical Collection, Detroit Public Library.)

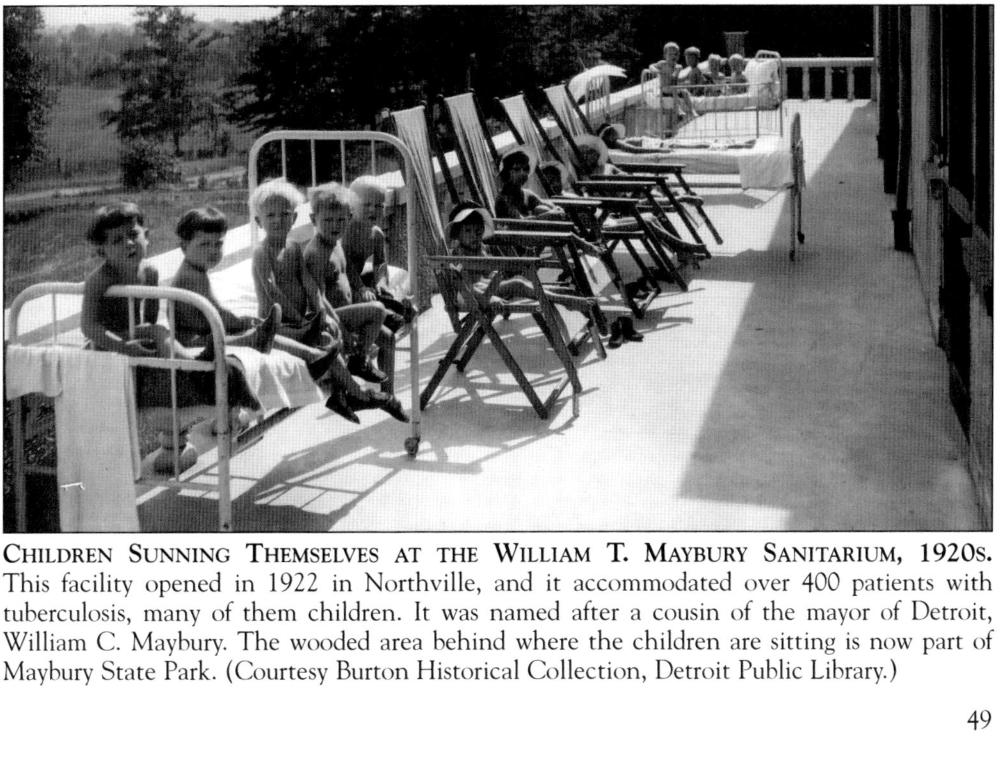

CHILDREN SUNNING THEMSELVES AT THE WILLIAM T. MAYBURY SANITARIUM, 1920S. This facility opened in 1922 in Northville, and it accommodated over 400 patients with tuberculosis, many of them children. It was named after a cousin of the mayor of Detroit, William C. Maybury. The wooded area behind where the children are sitting is now part of Maybury State Park. (Courtesy Burton Historical Collection, Detroit Public Library.)

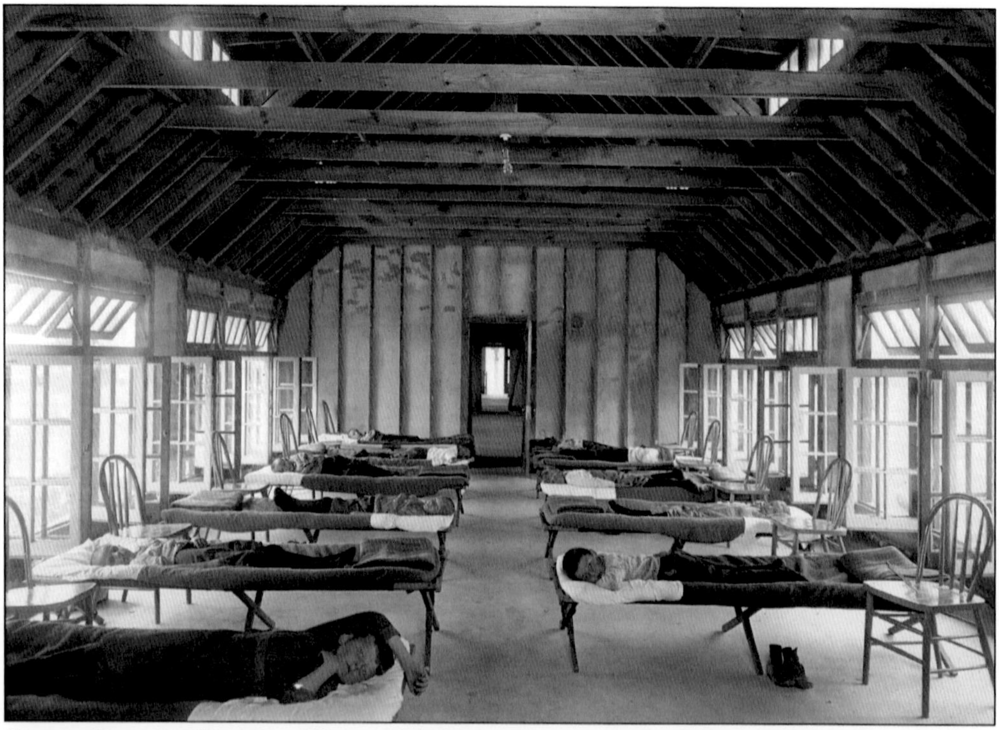

YOUNG BOYS IN SLEEPING WARDS, MAYBURY SANITARIUM, 1920S. These boys are resting on cots in a sleeping ward. The theory at the time was that fresh air and sunshine cured tuberculosis. In addition to patient wards, there were other buildings, such as a dining room building, a blacksmith shop, a garage, and a commissary. (Courtesy Burton Historical Collection, Detroit Public Library.)

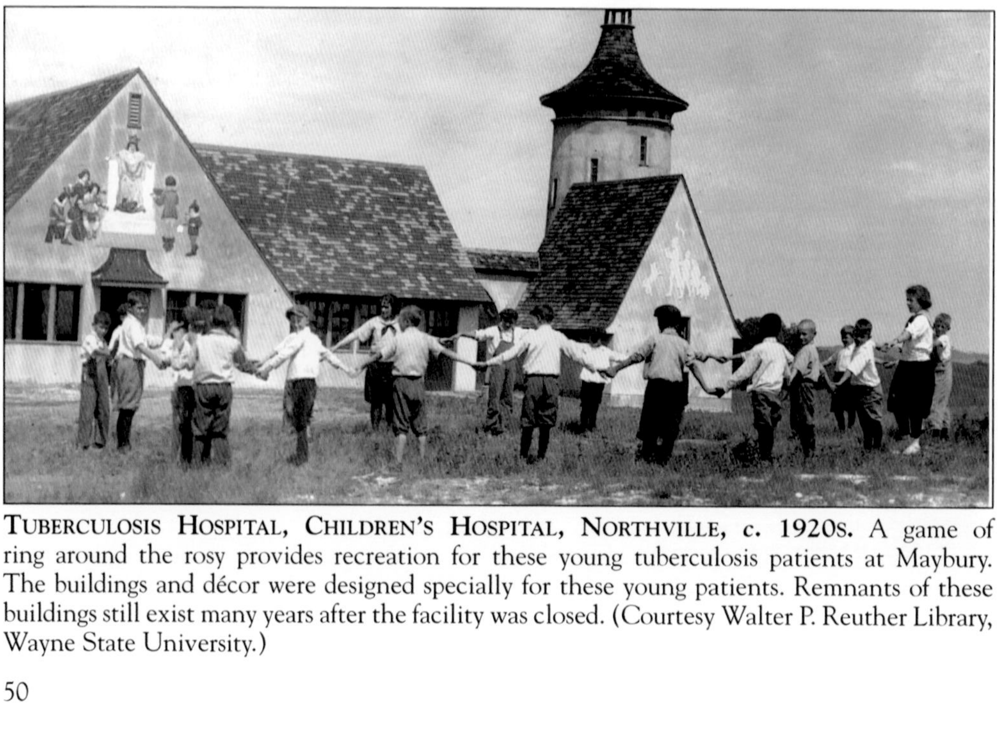

TUBERCULOSIS HOSPITAL, CHILDREN'S HOSPITAL, NORTHVILLE, c. 1920S. A game of ring around the rosy provides recreation for these young tuberculosis patients at Maybury. The buildings and décor were designed specially for these young patients. Remnants of these buildings still exist many years after the facility was closed. (Courtesy Walter P. Reuther Library, Wayne State University.)

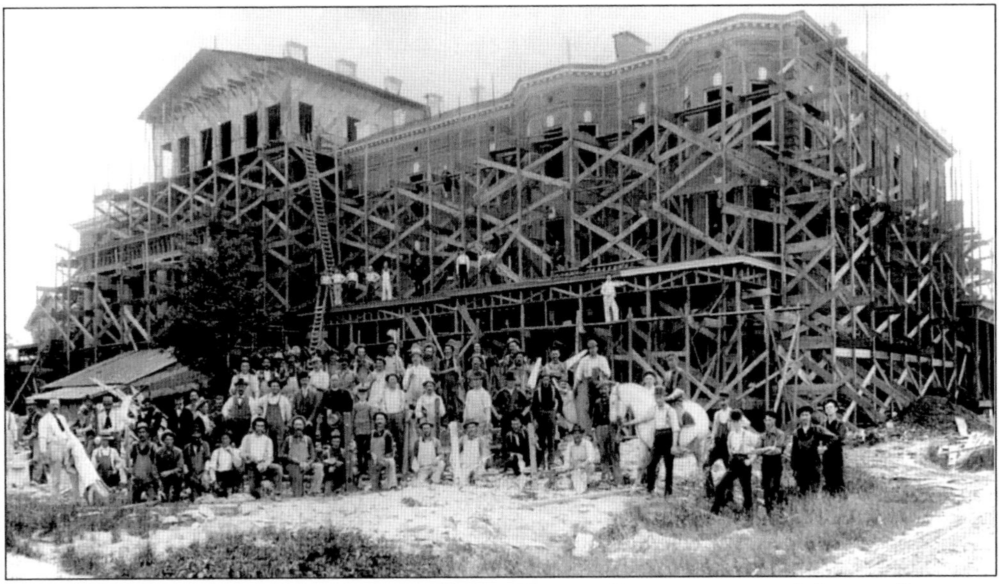

ST. JOSEPH'S SANITARIUM AND BATH HOUSE UNDER CONSTRUCTION, MOUNT CLEMENS, 1898. Work began on the new sanitarium and bath house November 4, 1898. Here the workers are taking a break to pose for a photograph. The architect was Theophilus Van Damme of Mount Clemens. The baths used heated mineral water that was pumped from 1,400 feet under the city. (Courtesy Archdiocese of Detroit.)

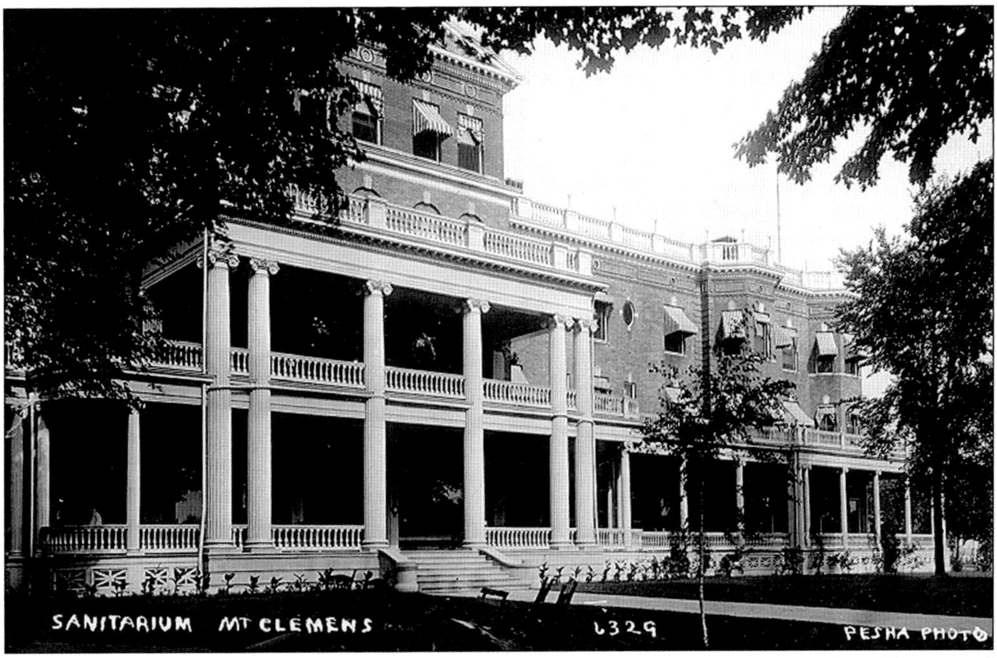

ST. JOSEPH'S SANITARIUM AND BATH HOUSE, MOUNT CLEMENS, c. 1910. This old postcard published by Pesha Publishing of Marine City, Michigan, is an exterior view of the sanitarium and bath house at 215 North Avenue. In 1900, a 50-bed hospital was opened on the third floor. This building still exists, and St. Joseph's Sanitarium evolved into the present St. Joseph's of Macomb. (Courtesy Mount Clemens Public Library.)

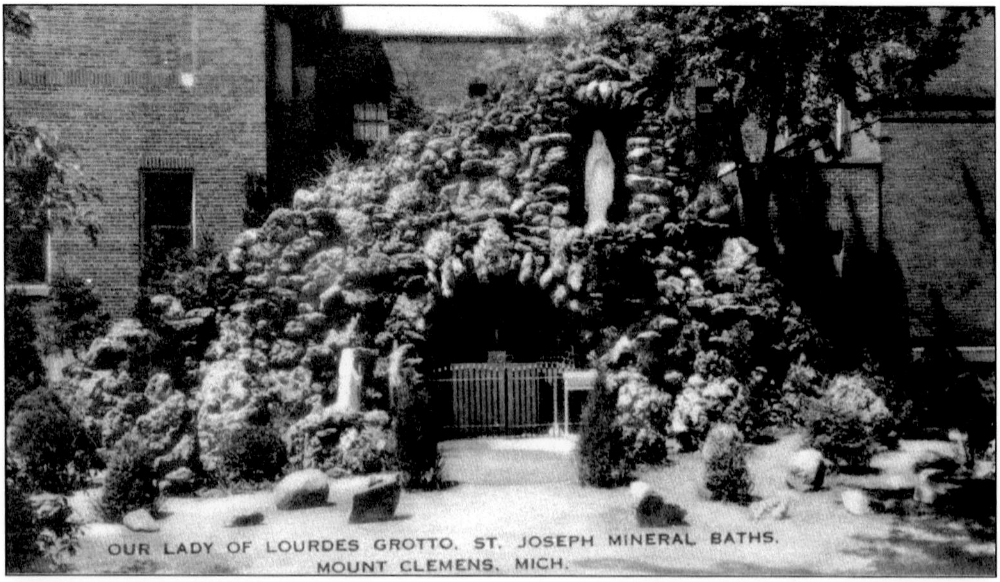

OUR LADY OF LOURDES GROTTO, ST. JOSEPH MINERAL BATHS, MOUNT CLEMENS. The Sisters of Charity of Mt. St. Joseph's, Cincinnati, Ohio, built this grotto at the mineral baths. The baths provided holistic therapy thought to cure everything from arthritis to eczema. Famous people such as Babe Ruth, Mae West, Jack Dempsey, William Randolph Hearst, and Henry Ford came to Mount Clemens for the baths. (Courtesy Archdiocese of Detroit.)

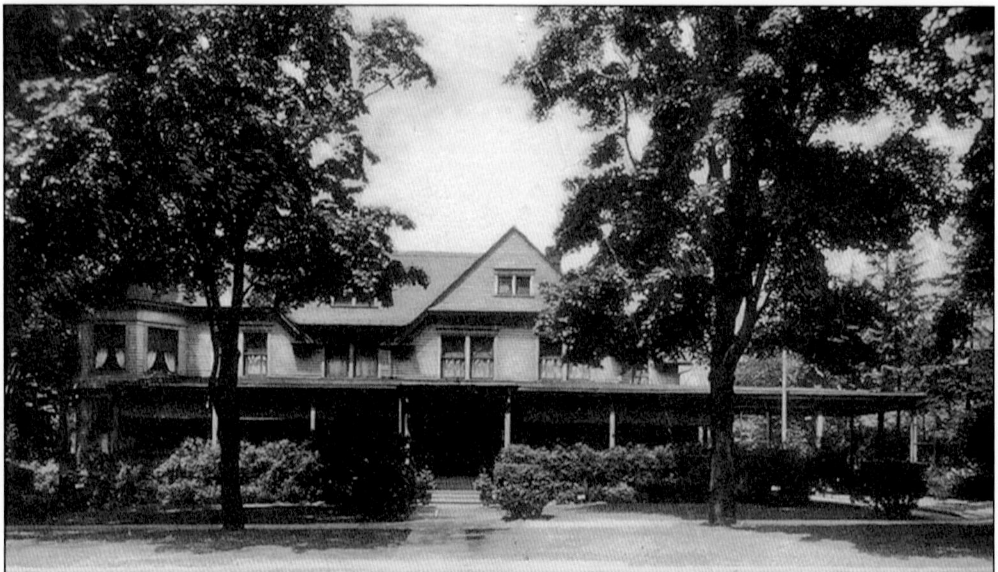

GRAY GABLES SANITARIUM, MOUNT CLEMENS, c. 1920. This sepia postcard shows the sanitarium that was located at 228 South Gratiot Avenue and operated by Dr. Enoch Mather from 1914 to 1947. Dr. Mather wrote that the sanitarium had plenty of windows, a beautiful veranda, and beautiful grounds laid out in a park with large shady trees. The building was later used as a retirement home until it burned in 1960. (Courtesy Mount Clemens Public Library.)

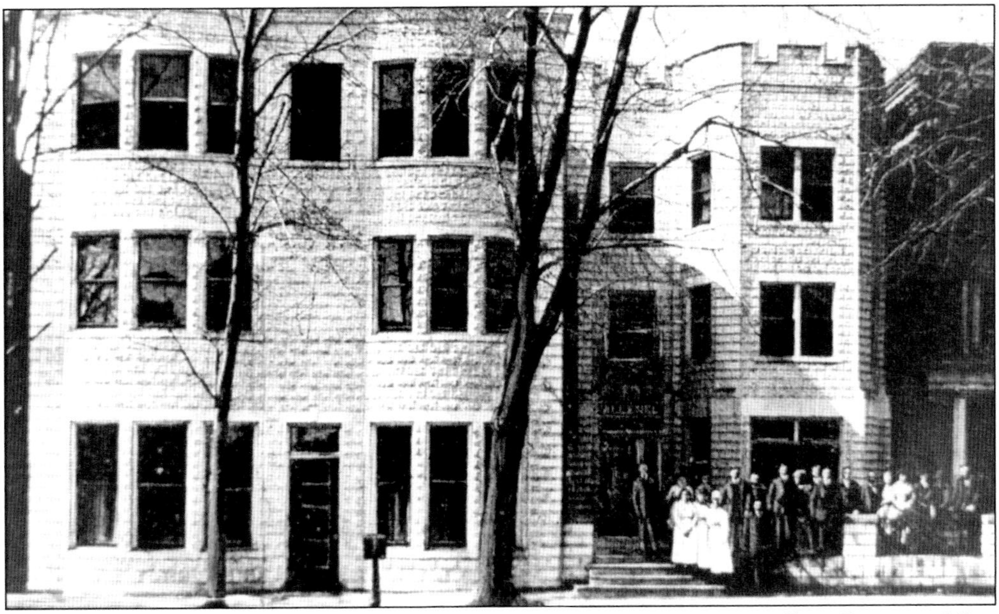

ALLENEL SANITARIUM AND STAFF, MOUNT CLEMENS, c. 1915. Dr. Albert Bertram Allen operated this sanitarium from 1912 until 1925. After that, it was Grace Hospital from 1926 to 1936, and was later used as apartments, first called the Allenel, and then the White Stone Apartments. The building was razed in 1978. (Courtesy Mount Clemens Public Library.)

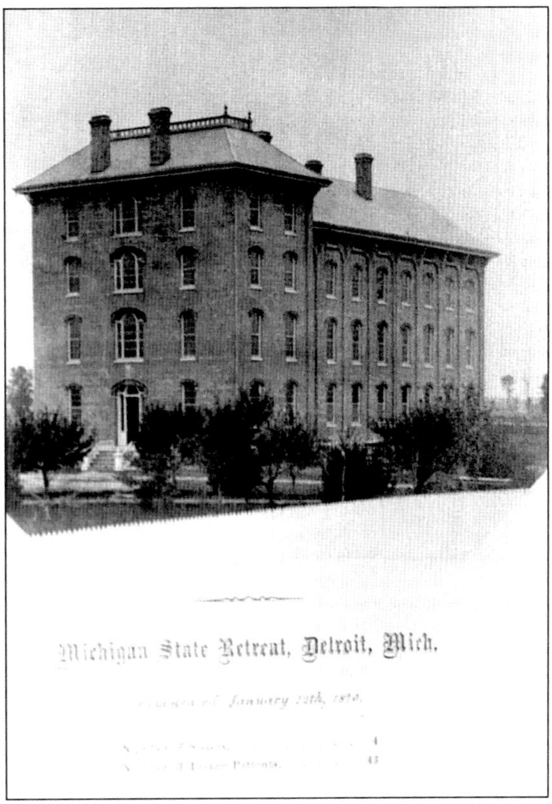

MICHIGAN RETREAT FOR THE INSANE, 1870. The Sisters of Charity opened this facility on Michigan Avenue and Twenty-forth Street in Detroit. This brick structure replaced the first frame structure in 1870. This facility housed 90 patients. It was renamed St. Joseph's Retreat in 1883. This was Michigan's first private mental hospital. (Courtesy Dearborn Historical Museum.)

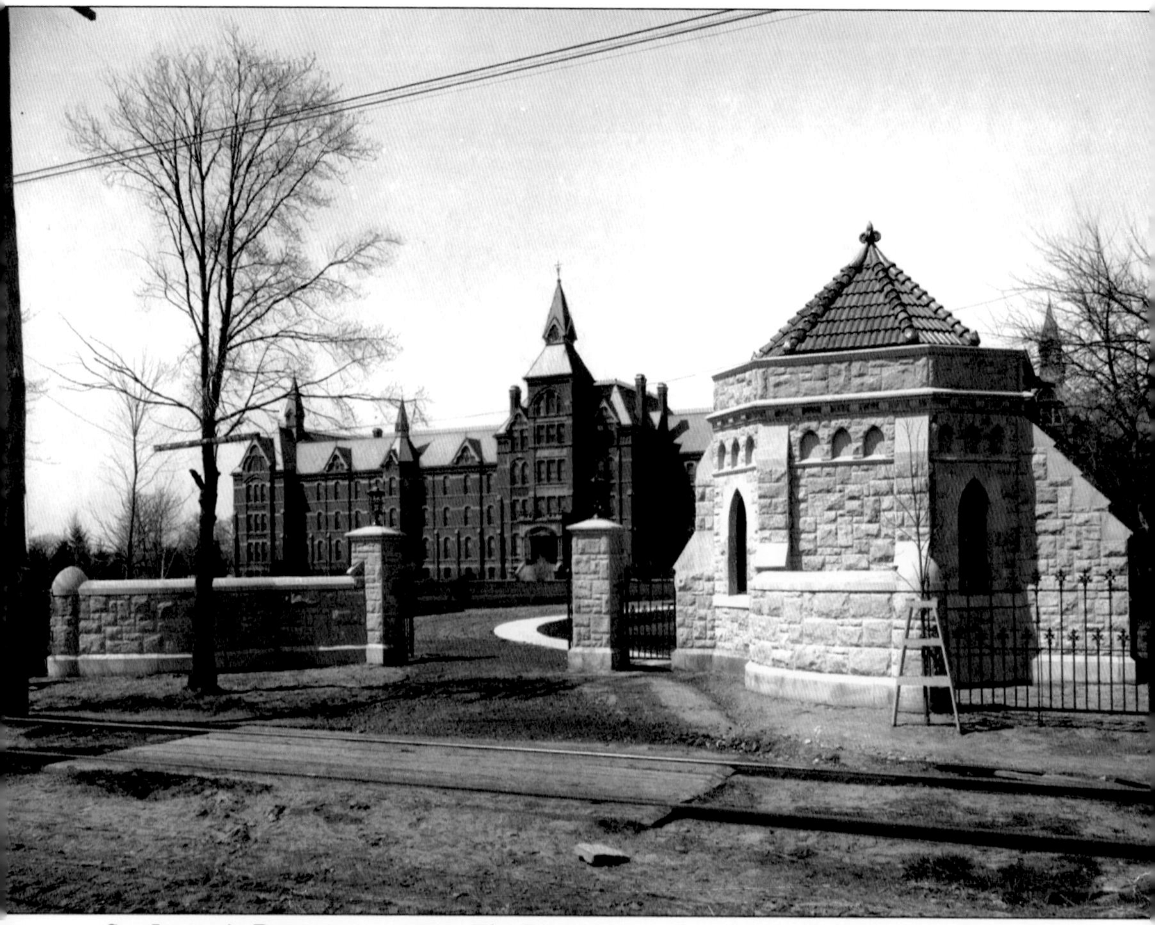

ST. JOSEPH'S RETREAT, c. 1920. The Retreat opened October 28, 1886, and this red brick Gothic Victorian building, surrounded by an iron fence, became a landmark in Dearborn. It was the first private mental institution in Michigan. It closed February 1, 1962, and the building was razed in 1963. All that is left to give evidence of its existence is a faded historic marker, which was dedicated May 21, 1974, at the now busy intersection of Outer Drive and Michigan Avenue in Dearborn. (Courtesy Daughters of Charity Archives, Mater Dei Provincialate, Evansville, Indiana.)

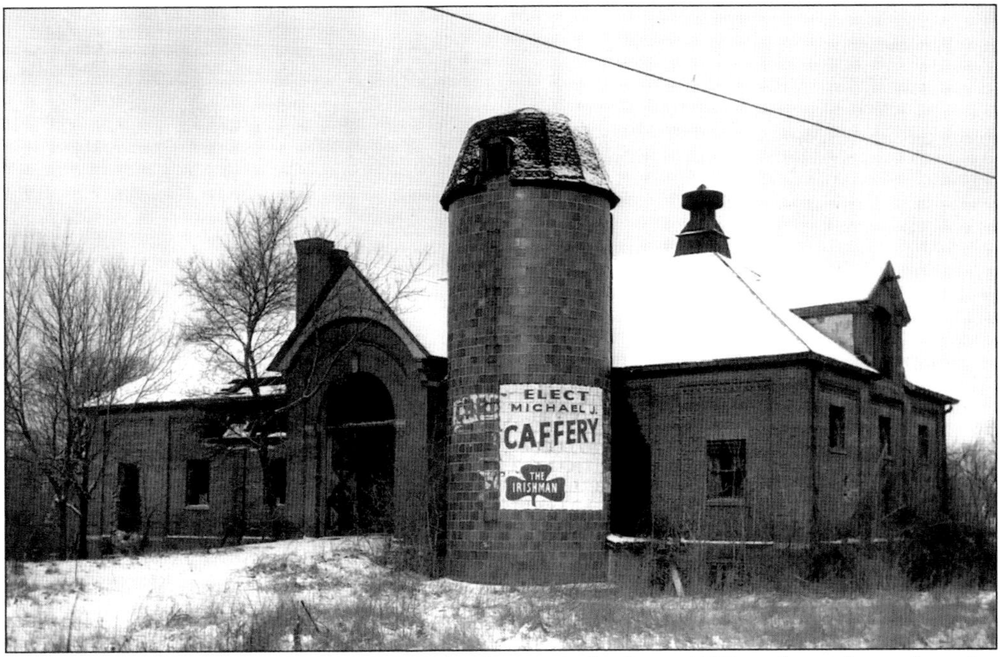

ST. JOSEPH'S RETREAT BARN, 1958. The barn was built in 1887 and was located at the northwest corner of Michigan and Outer Drive. It was used to house cattle and horses and to store feed until 1945. The photo was taken January 30, 1958, just before it was demolished. The Village Plaza mall is now on that site. (Courtesy Dearborn Historical Museum.)

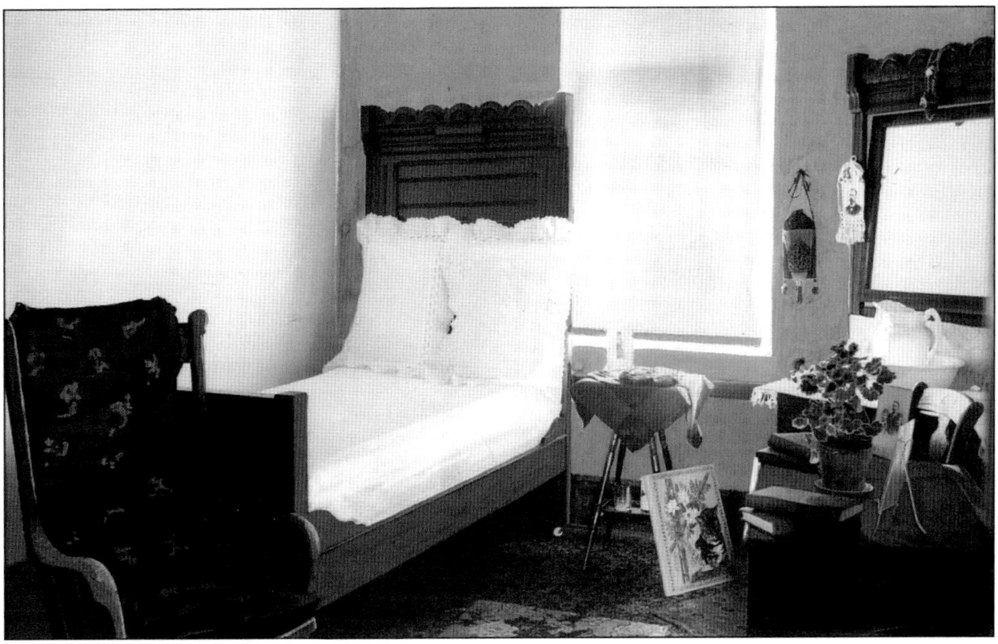

PATIENT'S BEDROOM, ST. JOSEPH'S RETREAT. This photo was in the 1893 Annual Report. Originally the building could accommodate 175, but wings were added in 1887 and 1896 which brought the total number of patients the Retreat could accommodate to 400. (Courtesy Dearborn Historical Museum.)

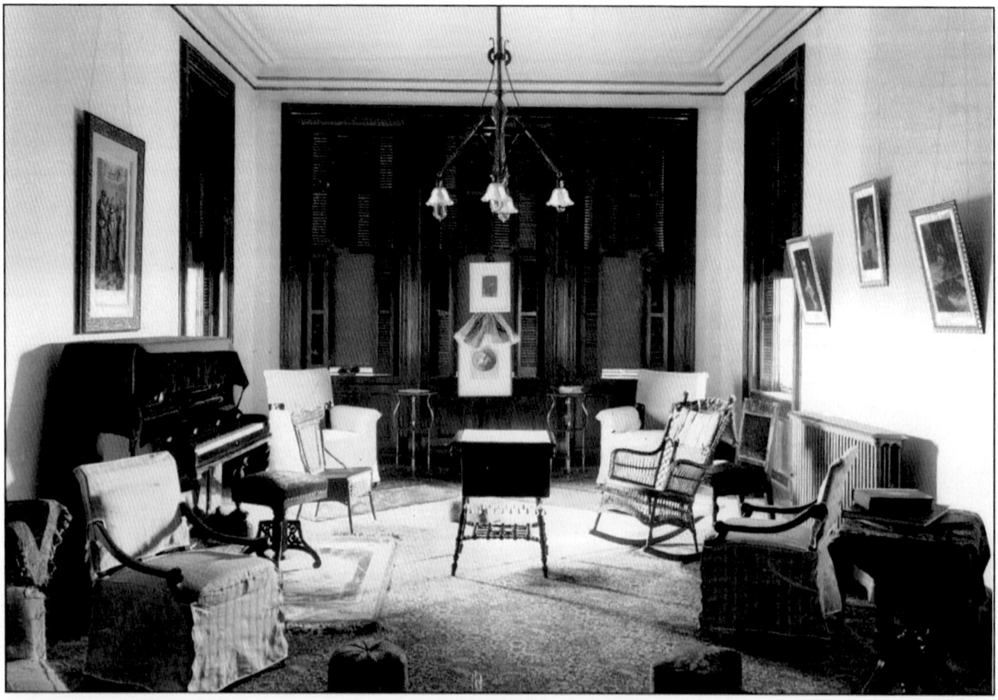

PATIENT'S PRIVATE PARLOR, ST. JOSEPH'S RETREAT, 1893. This photo of a private parlor on the second floor was included in the twelfth annual report of the institution, and shows the beautiful furnishings provided for the patients. The rooms were furnished with rich rugs, lace curtains, and mahogany and walnut furniture. (Courtesy Dearborn Historical Museum.)

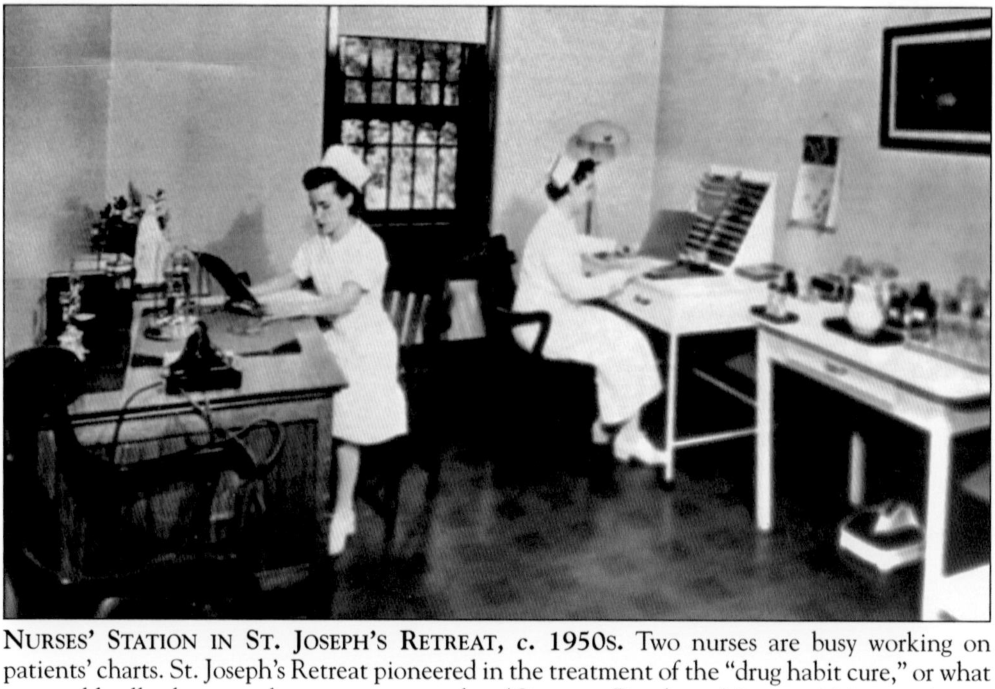

NURSES' STATION IN ST. JOSEPH'S RETREAT, c. 1950S. Two nurses are busy working on patients' charts. St. Joseph's Retreat pioneered in the treatment of the "drug habit cure," or what we would call substance abuse treatment today. (Courtesy Dearborn Historical Museum.)

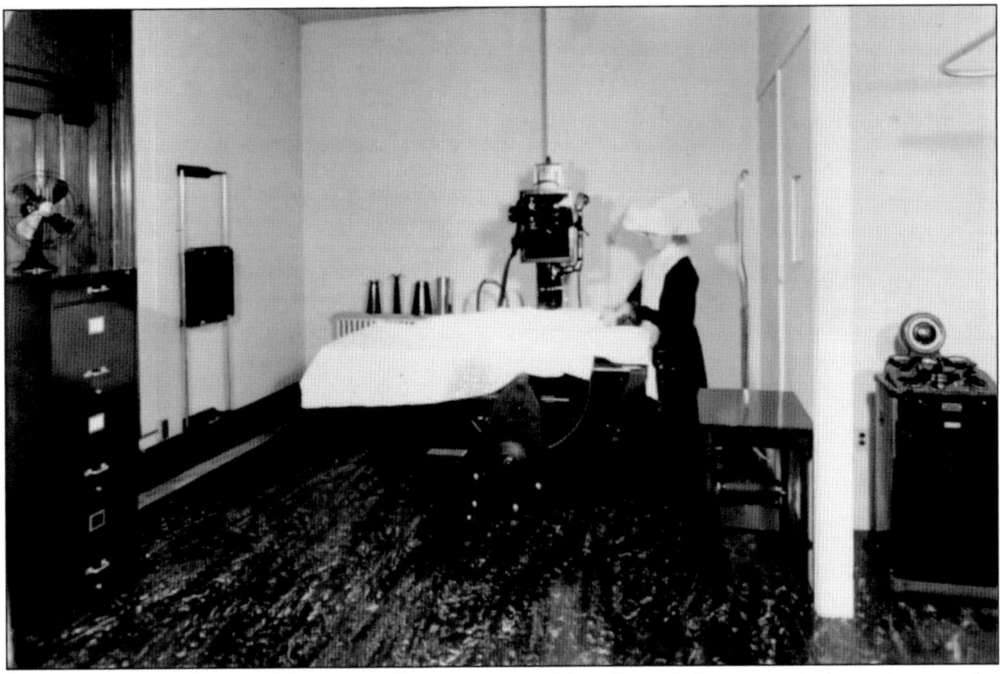

X-RAY DEPARTMENT, ST. JOSEPH'S RETREAT, c. 1950. One of the sisters is preparing to take an x-ray of a patient. The hospital also had a laboratory to do blood tests. (Courtesy Daughters of Charity Archives, Mater Dei Provincialate, Evansville, Indiana.)

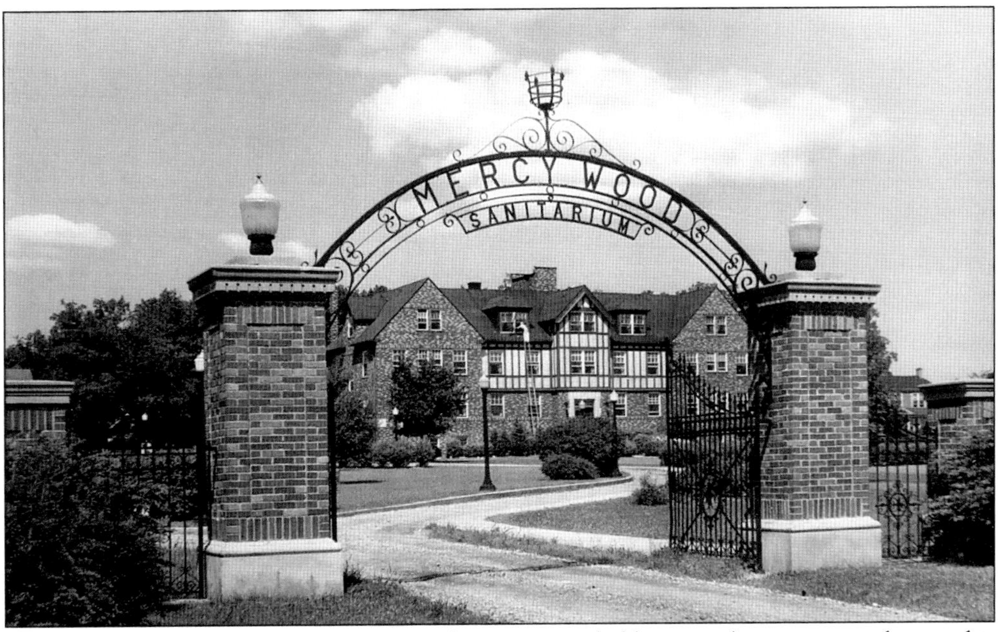

MERCYWOOD HOSPITAL, ANN ARBOR. The man on a ladder is working on a window at this private mental hospital which was run by the Sisters of Mercy. It was built in 1924, and was located on 80 acres of land on Jackson Road two miles west of Ann Arbor. It closed in 1986, and a new facility was opened on the Huron River Drive Campus. This building was demolished. (Courtesy Sisters of Mercy Archives, Farmington, Michigan.)

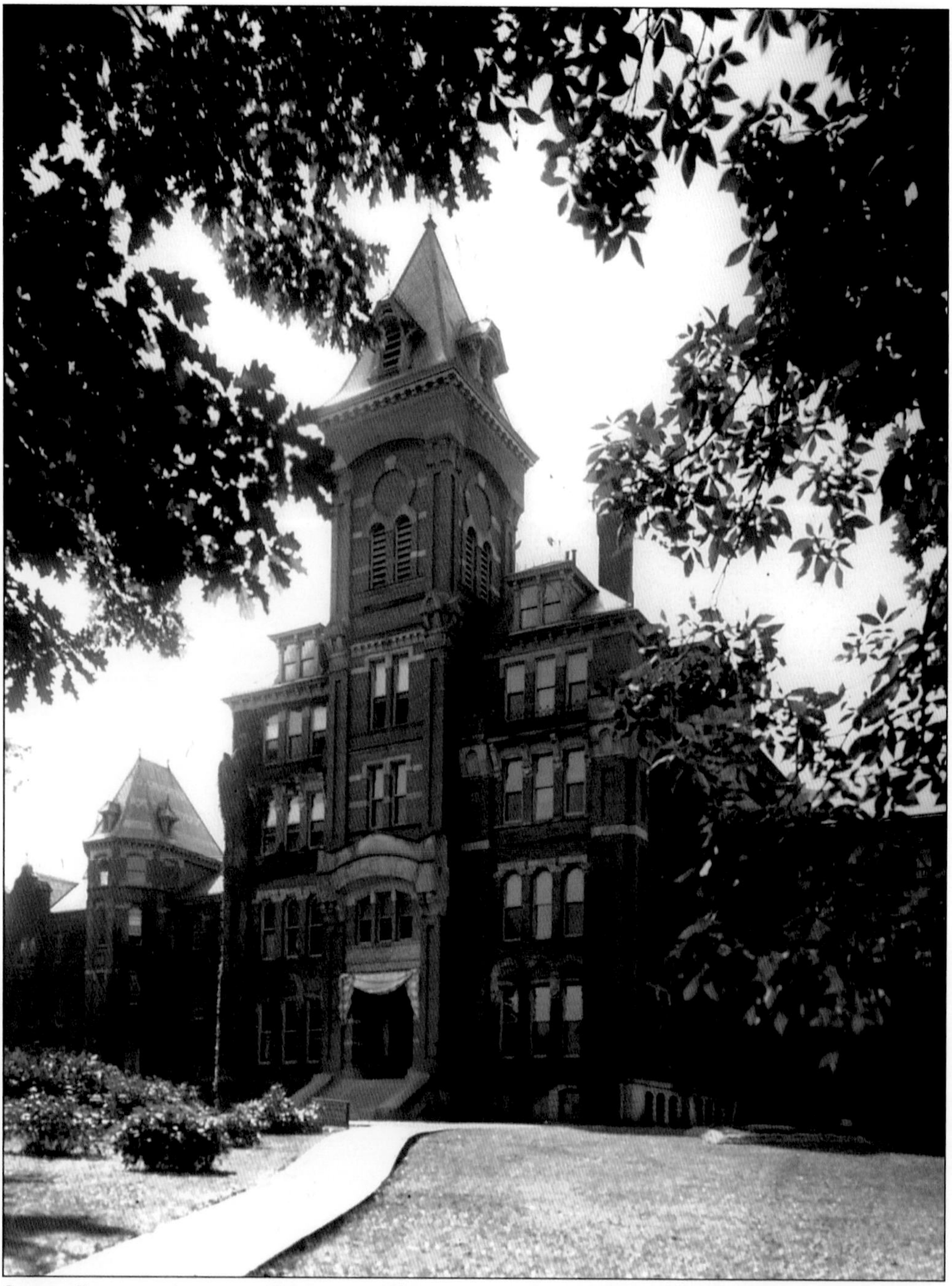

State Insane Asylum, Pontiac. This is an undated photograph of the administration building which was part of the large complex originally called the Eastern Michigan Asylum when it was built in 1878. It was renamed the Clinton Valley Center in 1973, and at one time had over 3,000 patients. It was added to the National Register of Historic Places in 1981 and was described as among the "most architecturally distinguished High Victorian Gothic structures in Michigan." That designation failed to save it from the wrecking ball in the year 2000. (Courtesy Walter P. Reuther Library, Wayne State University.)

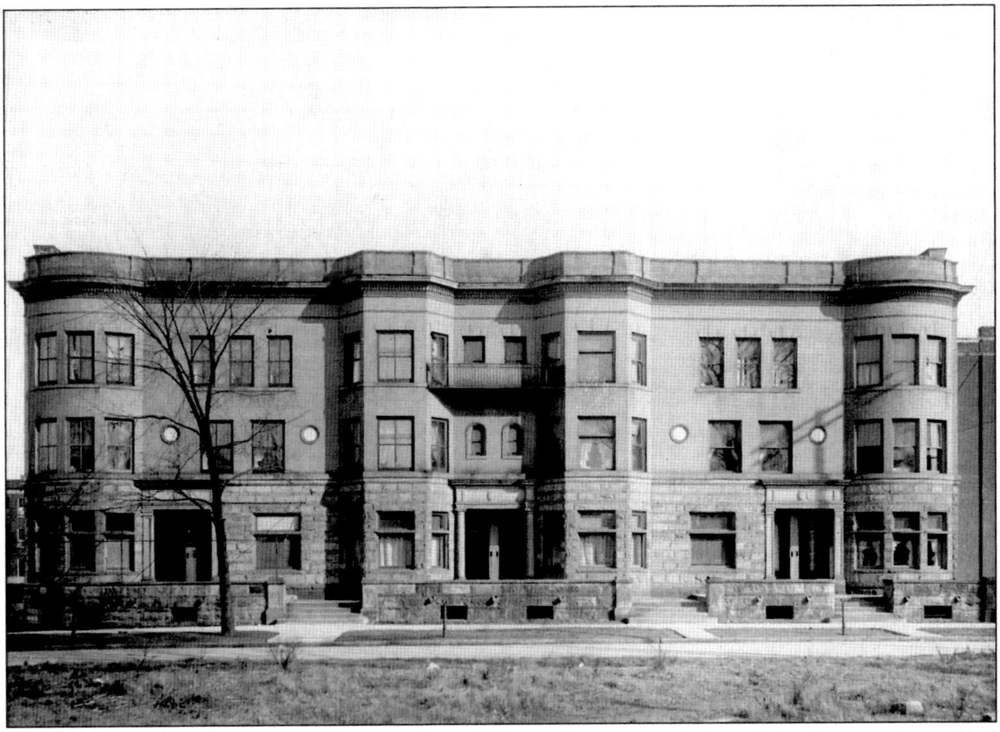

KING HOSPITAL, c. 1920. This was another of Detroit's many small hospitals that was also called King's Hospital for the Insane. It was located at 1006–1010 Brush, and B. Horton Barr, M.D., was the superintendent in 1911. (Courtesy Burton Historical Collection, Detroit Public Library.)

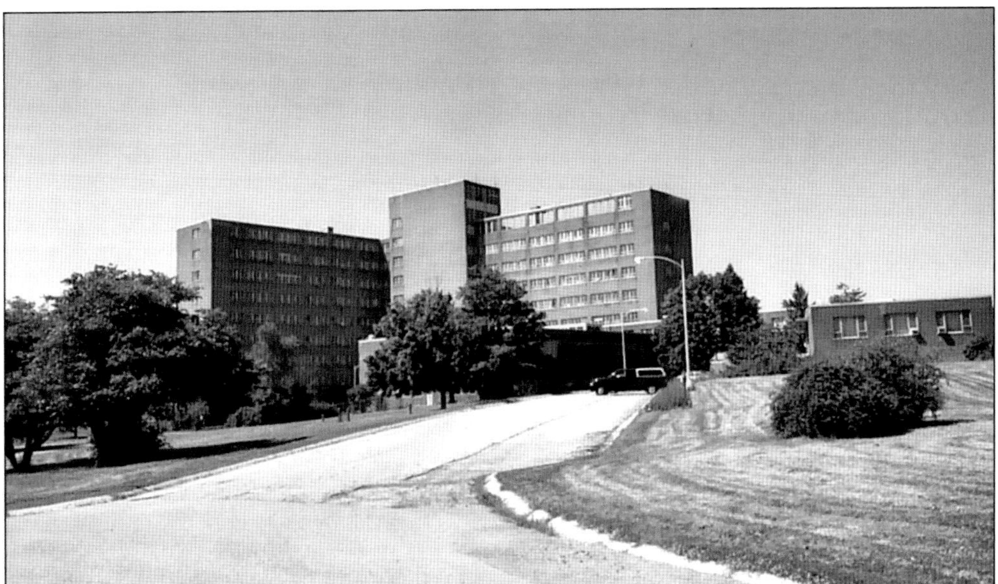

NORTHVILLE STATE HOSPITAL, 2003. Vacant and awaiting demolition, this state mental hospital was built in the 1950s and housed 300 patients, including children. It was also called Northville Regional Psychiatric Hospital. The prime 400 acres of wooded real estate will be sold to developers, no doubt to become the site of luxury condominiums.

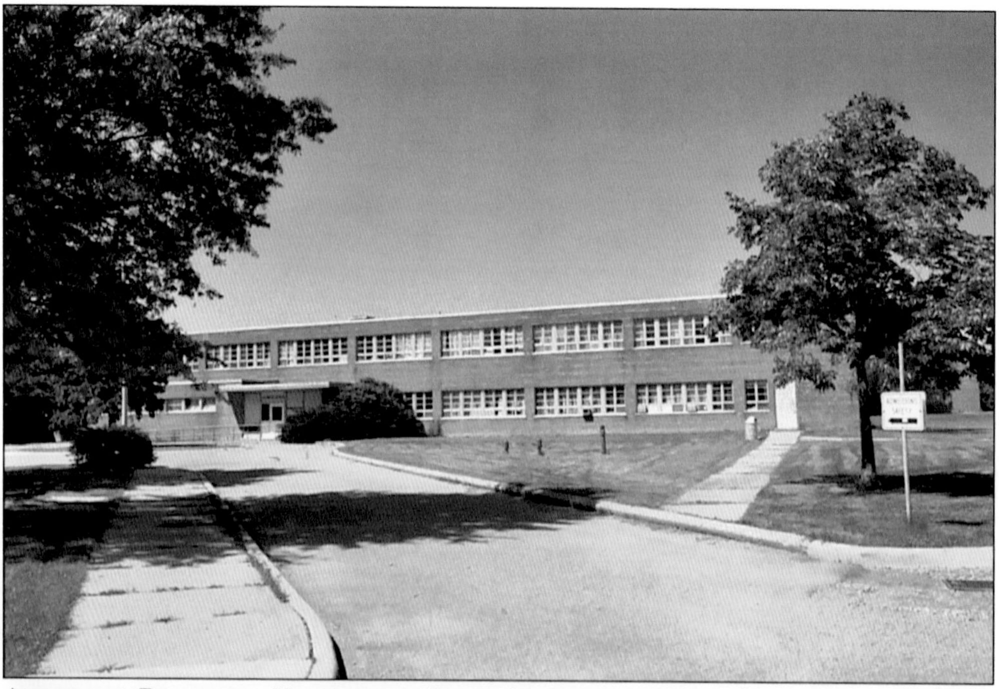

ADMISSION BUILDING, NORTHVILLE STATE HOSPITAL, 2003. This building is one of several on the grounds of the former state mental hospital. At one time it was a very busy place, but it now sits empty.

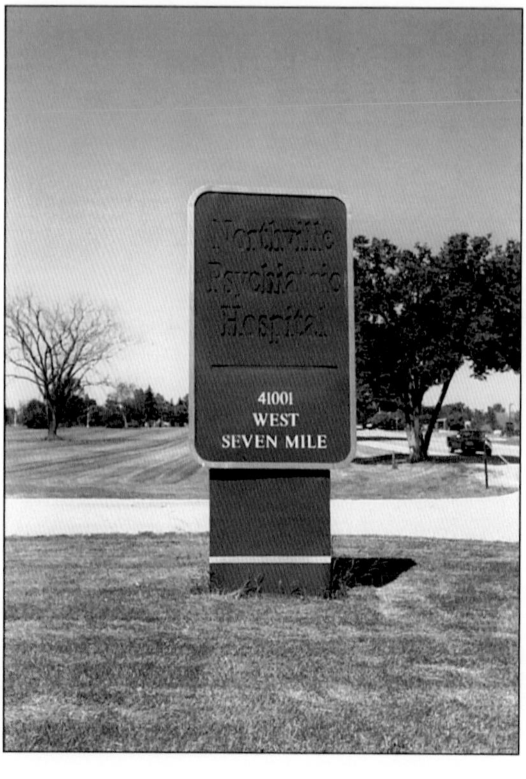

SIGN AT ENTRANCE TO NORTHVILLE STATE HOSPITAL, 2003. The address is still on the sign at the entrance of Northville State, but the paint from the words "Northville Psychiatric Hospital" has been removed.

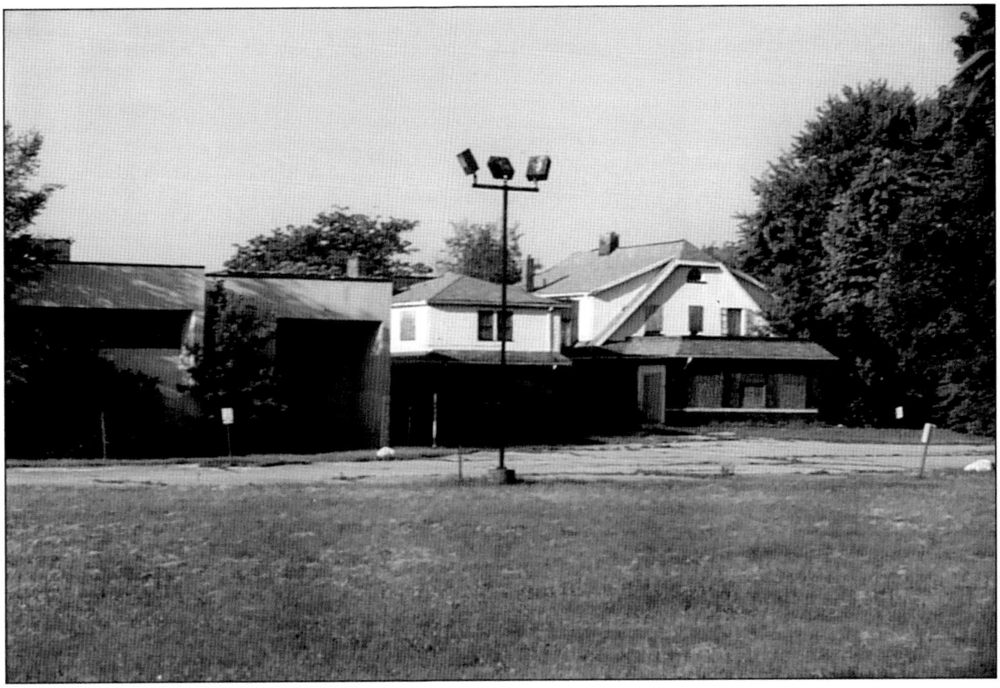

ARDMORE ACRES PSYCHIATRIC HOSPITAL, 2003. Ardmore, built in 1926 as a private psychiatric hospital, sat vacant and boarded up for ten years after it closed in 1993. There were some, mainly teenagers, who considered the building haunted and full of ghosts. These photos were taken shortly before it was razed in October of 2003. The 25 acres of land in Livonia, on Farmington Road between 7 and 8 Mile, is destined to become the site of condominiums. (Courtesy *Gazette* Newspapers.)

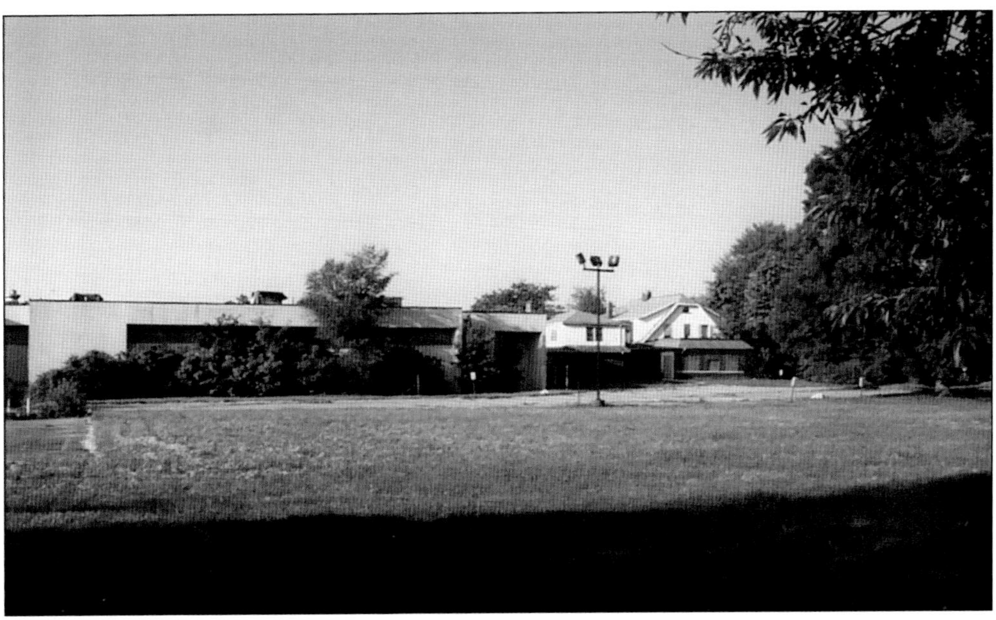

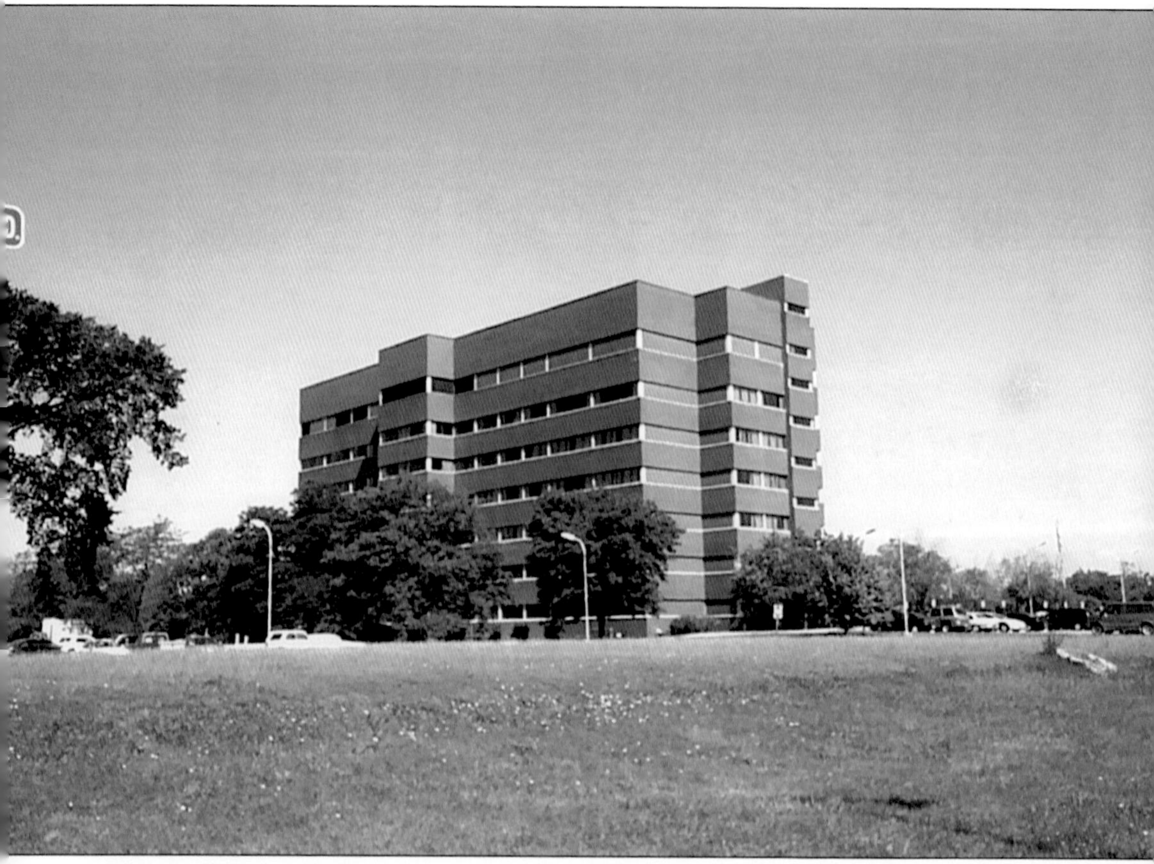

WALTER P. REUTHER PSYCHIATRIC FACILITY, 2003. This building was built in 1974 as part of the Wayne County General Hospital complex, and was used to house chronically ill patients. It is now one of the few inpatient psychiatric facilities still run by the State of Michigan. It was named to honor Walter P. Reuther, a fiery visionary of economic and social reform who built the United Automobile Workers (UAW) into one of the most militant and progressive unions in American history. He was an unceasing fighter for civil rights, improved health care, affordable housing, and the environment.

Three

Eloise

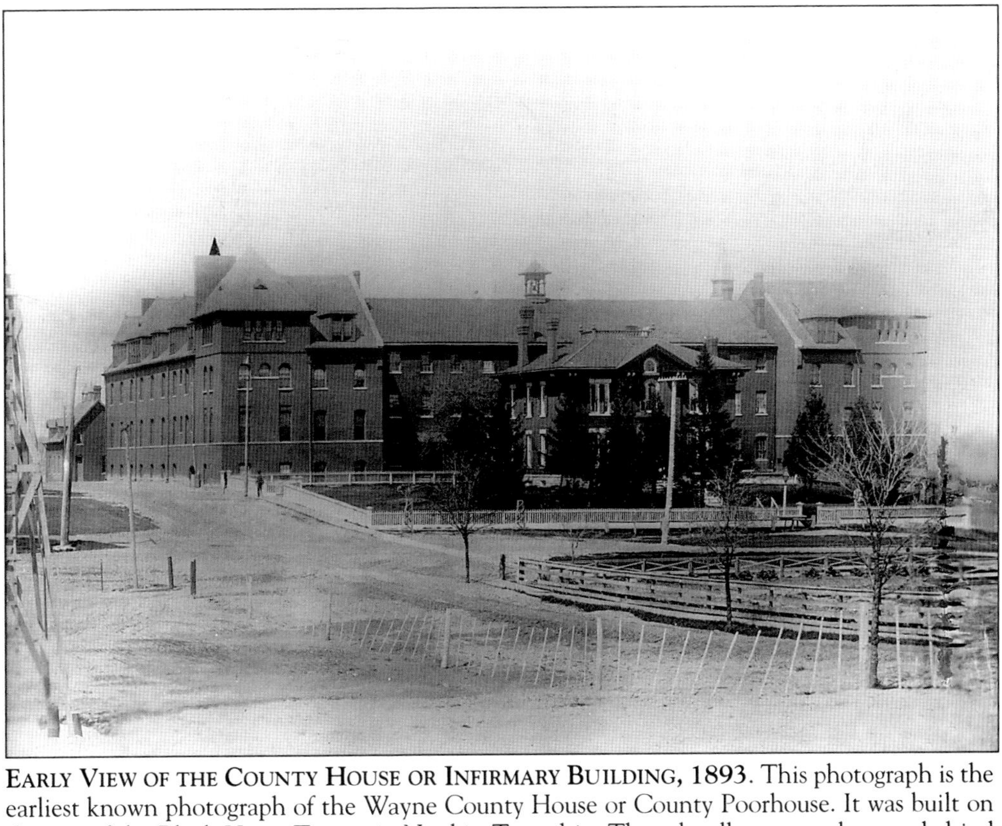

Early View of the County House or Infirmary Building, 1893. This photograph is the earliest known photograph of the Wayne County House or County Poorhouse. It was built on the site of the Black Horse Tavern in Nankin Township. The schoolhouse can be seen behind the main building, and part of a windmill used to pump water from the artificial lake is to the left. (Courtesy Eloise Museum, Westland, Michigan.)

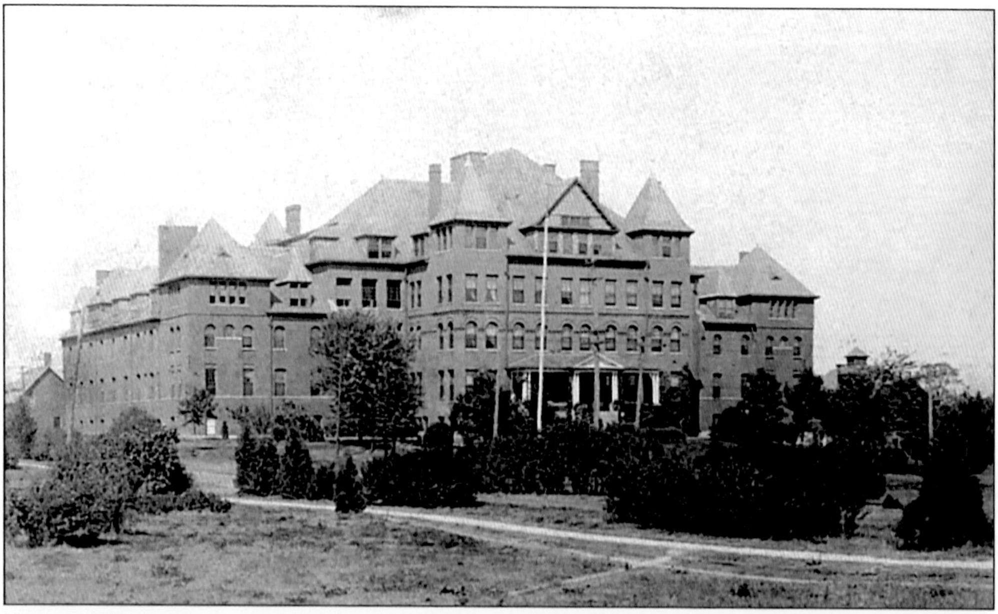

ELOISE, MICHIGAN, c. 1906. This rare black and white Eloise penny postcard was postmarked November 10, 1906. It was sent to Miss Lottie Wright of Three Oaks, Michigan. The notation on the side of the card is "show Hettie where Edith works. Cecil." The hospital was a major employer in Wayne County, and many employees lived on the grounds. (Courtesy Eloise Museum, Westland, Michigan.)

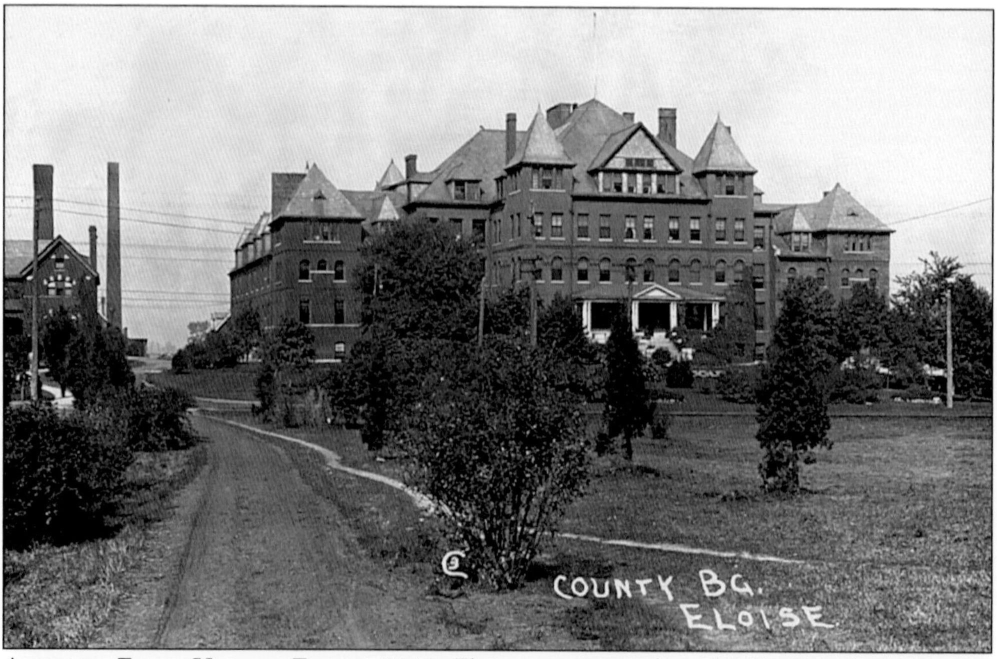

ANOTHER EARLY VIEW OF ELOISE, 1910. Eloise was captured on this black and white penny postcard that was postmarked January 27, 1910, and sent to Miss Anna M. Hess of Rome, New York. The writer stated that he lived in the building to the left which was the administration building. The smokestacks from the power plant are visible in the background.

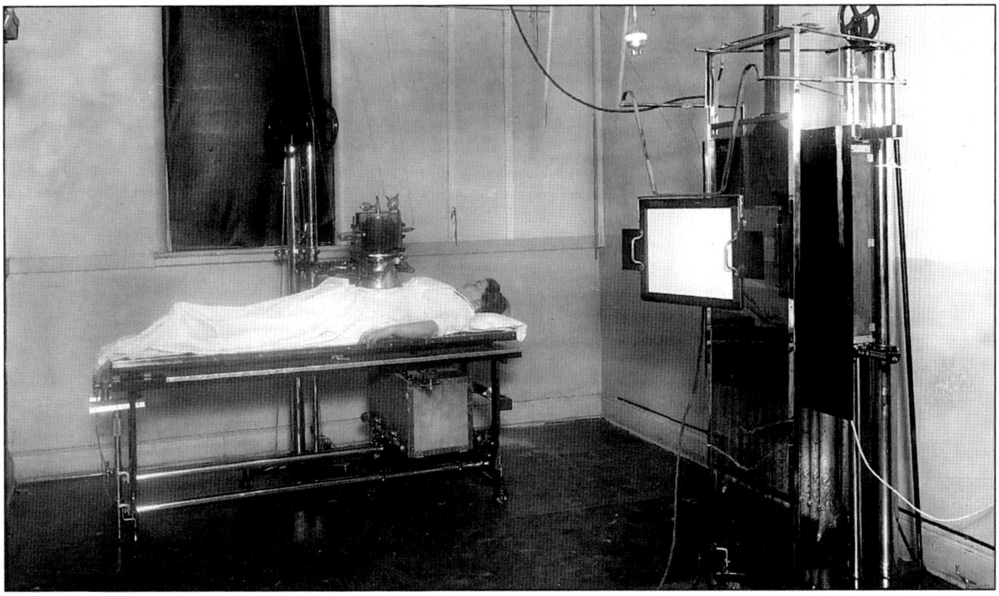

First X-rays, c. 1915. Eloise was among the first, if not the first, hospital to use x-rays to diagnose patients. The Infirmary Building had an x-ray machine, and patients came from Detroit and other communities to have x-rays taken. This woman is receiving an x-ray of her abdomen. (Courtesy Eloise Museum, Westland, Michigan.)

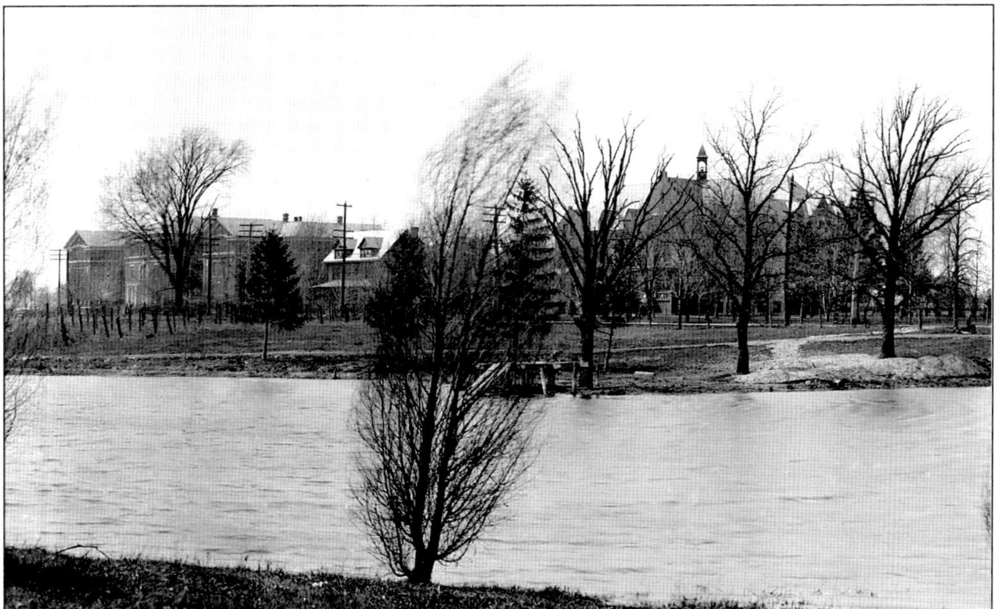

Eloise Grounds, 1919. This windswept, wintry view across the artificial lake shows hospital building "D" (name later changed to Building "G" in 1932), the double residence which was home to the hospital superintendent, and hospital building "E" (name later changed to Building "H" in 1932.) The double residence was built in 1895, and was first occupied by Dr. E.O. Bennett, the superintendent, and Mr. Stanislas Keenan, the chief clerk and bookkeeper. (Courtesy Eloise Museum, Westland, Michigan.)

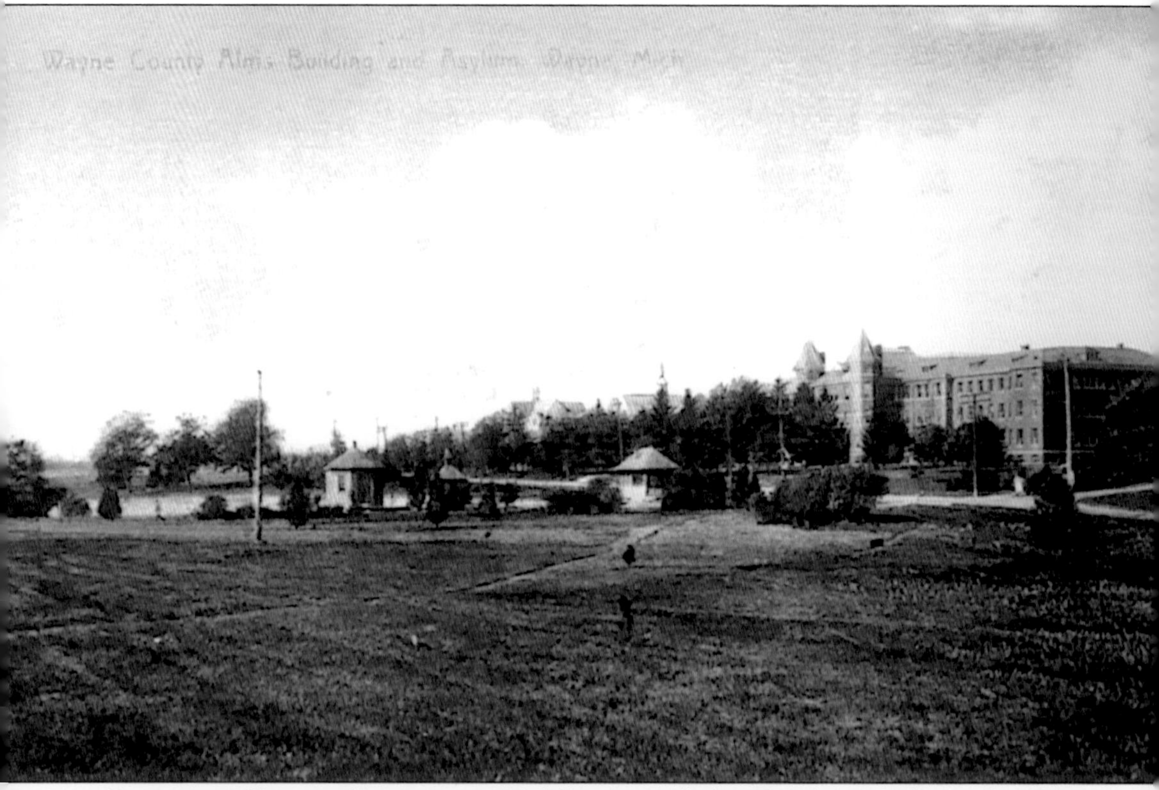

PANORAMIC VIEW OF ELOISE, c. 1895. This postcard identifies this complex as the Wayne County Alms Building and incorrectly places it in Wayne, Michigan, when it was actually located in Nankin Township, now Westland. The Asylum building is on the left and the Wayne

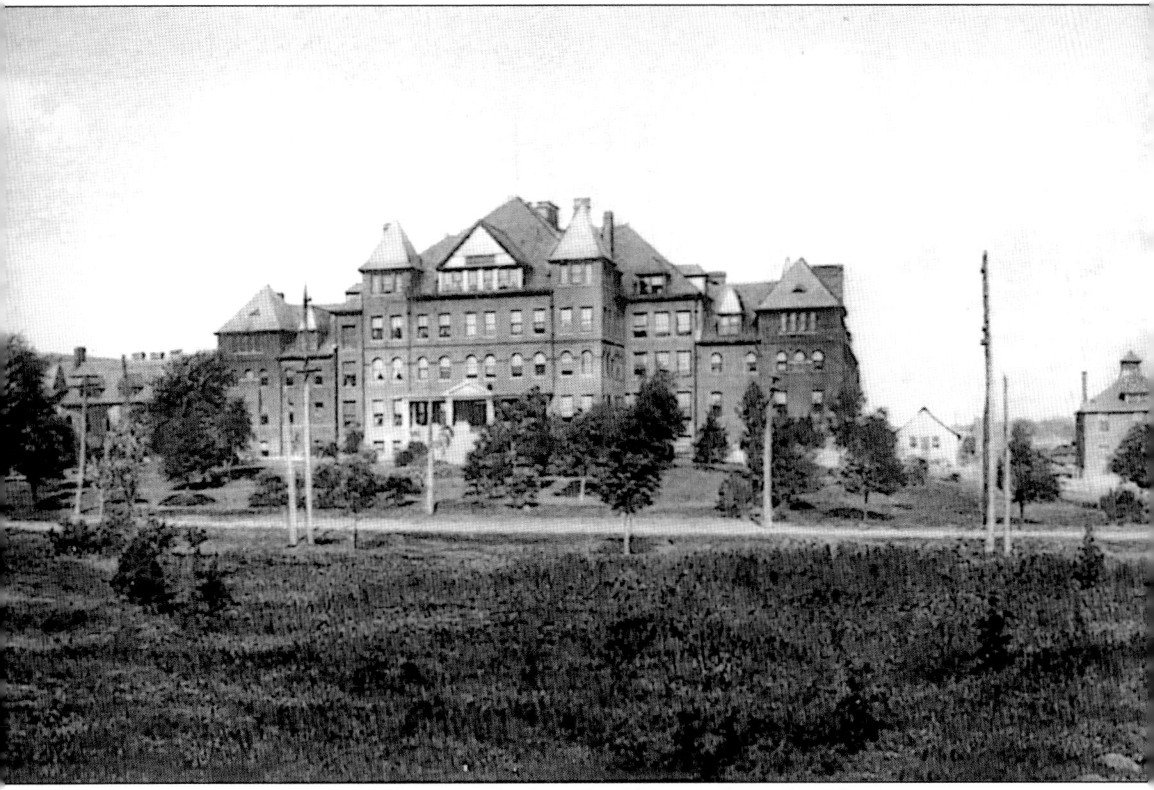

County House or County Poorhouse is the large building to the right. The water tower is in between the two buildings. (Courtesy Dearborn Historical Museum.)

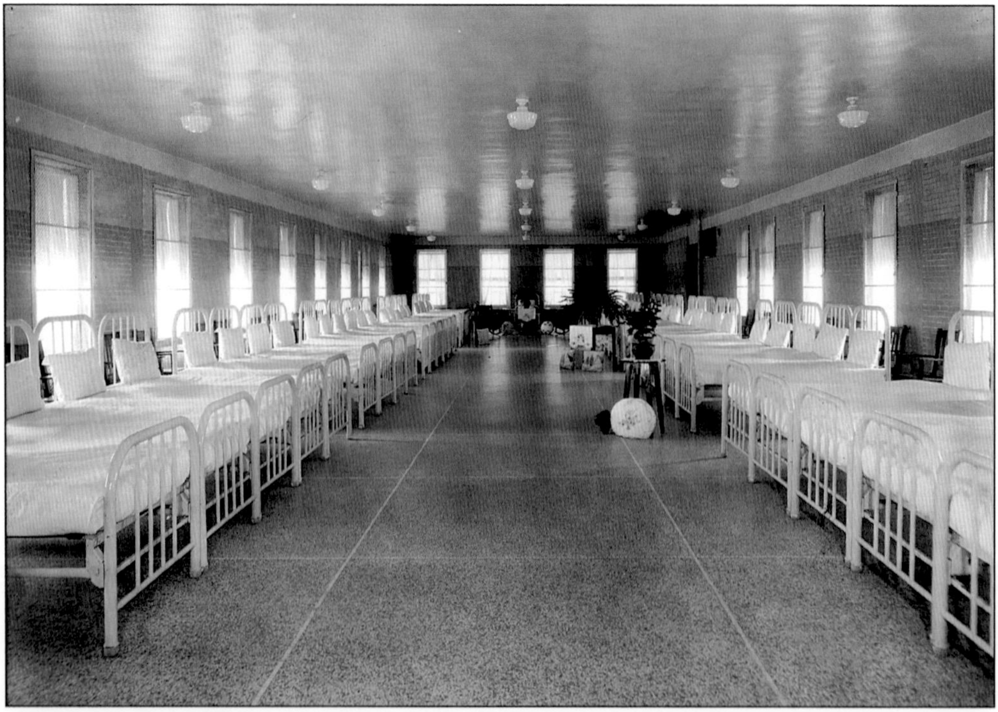

A Patient Ward, Building "I," c. 1922. This photo was probably taken when the building first opened in 1922. It was used to house 240 female psychiatric patients in large, open wards. Each patient had a bed and a chair. This building was one of six similar buildings that were vacated in 1973 when patients were transferred to state psychiatric hospitals. (Courtesy Eloise Museum, Westland, Michigan.)

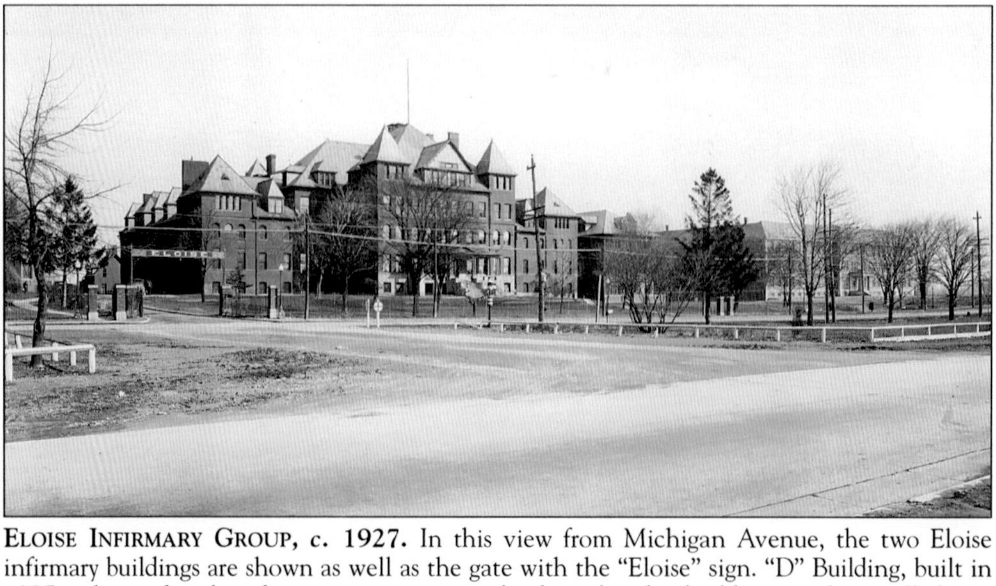

Eloise Infirmary Group, c. 1927. In this view from Michigan Avenue, the two Eloise infirmary buildings are shown as well as the gate with the "Eloise" sign. "D" Building, built in 1925 to house female infirmary patients, is at the far right; this building was later called "A" Building. The building to the right of the Eloise sign was remodeled to create the William J. Seymour Hospital in 1933. (Courtesy Eloise Museum, Westland, Michigan.)

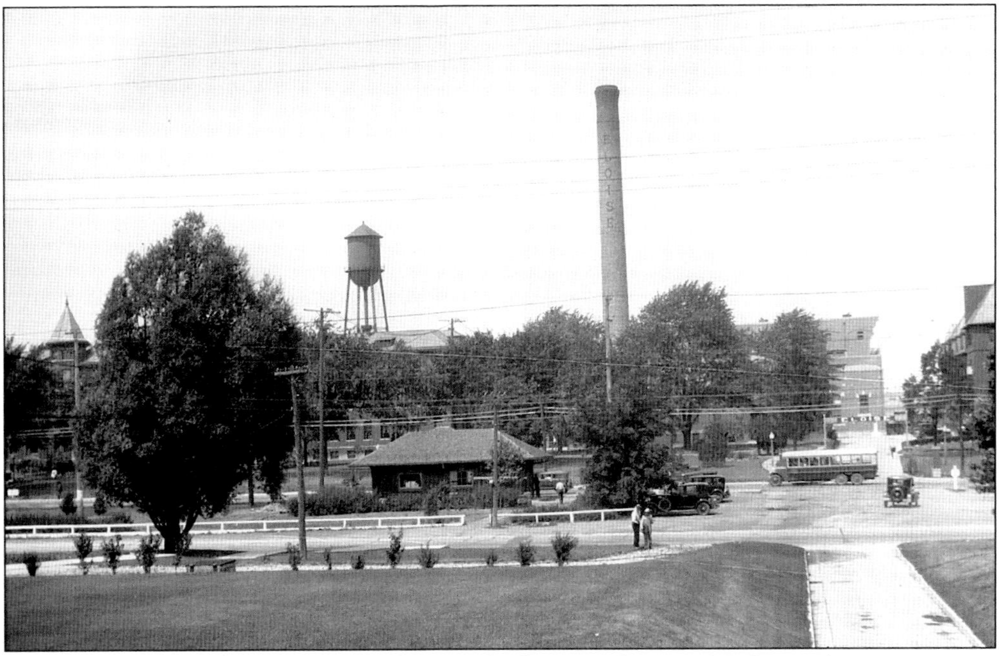

ENTRANCE TO ELOISE, c. 1929. In this view looking north across Michigan Avenue, one can see the trolley station, a bus passing the gate into Eloise, the Eloise smokestack, and the water tower. The power plant is visible beyond the gate, and the Infirmary Building can be partially seen to the right of the gate. (Courtesy Eloise Museum, Westland, Michigan.)

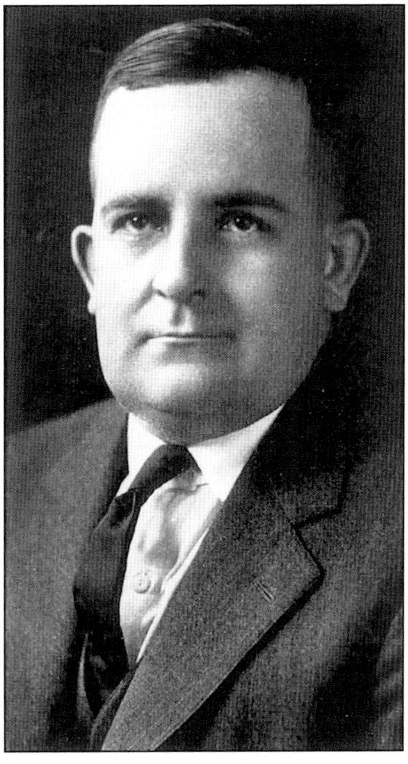

THOMAS REUBEN KELLER GRUBER, M.D., SUPERINTENDENT OF ELOISE, 1929–1949. Dr. Gruber came to Eloise from Detroit Receiving Hospital, and was the superintendent at the institution during a period of rapid growth when the patient population reached 10,000. (Courtesy Eloise Museum, Westland, Michigan.)

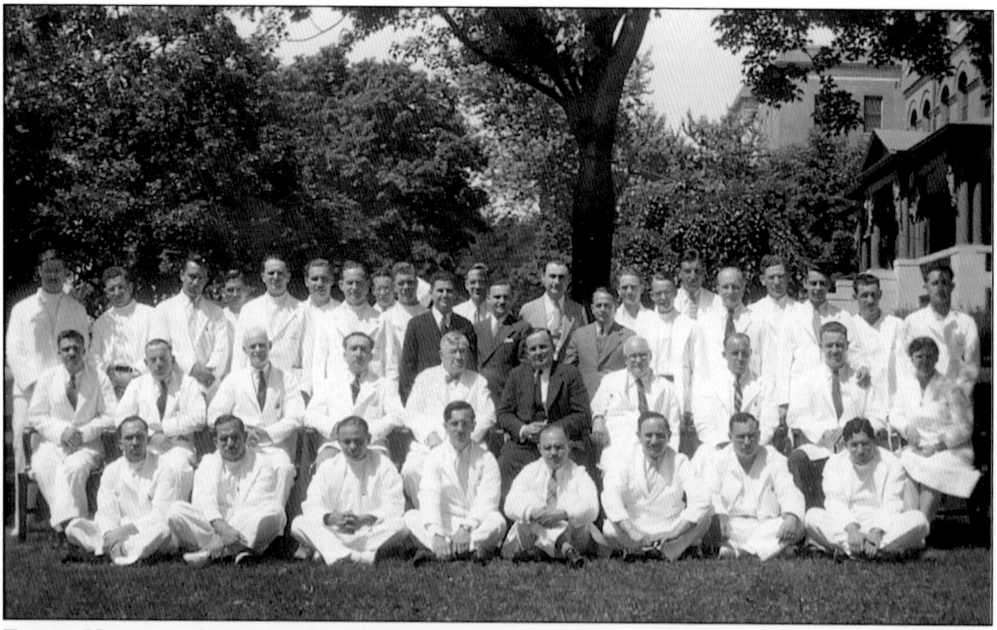

ELOISE HOSPITAL STAFF, 1934–1935. Thomas K. Gruber, general superintendent of Eloise, is seated in the center wearing a business suit in the midst of the medical staff of the general hospital and psychiatric division. This photograph was taken on the lawn in front of the William J. Seymour General Hospital at Eloise, Michigan. (Courtesy Eloise Museum, Westland, Michigan.)

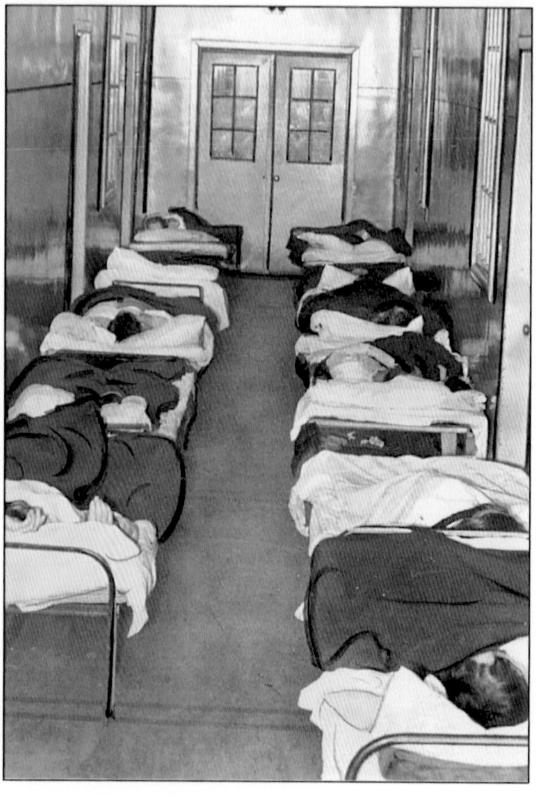

OVERCROWDED CONDITIONS, BUILDING "F," c. 1940S. Patients are lined up on cots in hallways in what was originally called the Women's New Building which was built in 1893 and razed in 1955. The building was designed to house 170 women, but it was overflowing with patients when this photo was taken. (Courtesy Eloise Museum, Westland, Michigan.)

HALLWAY, PSYCHIATRIC BUILDING, c. 1940S. An empty hallway provides a glimpse of what the inside of the psychiatric buildings looked like to employees and visitors who used them. (Courtesy Eloise Museum, Westland, Michigan.)

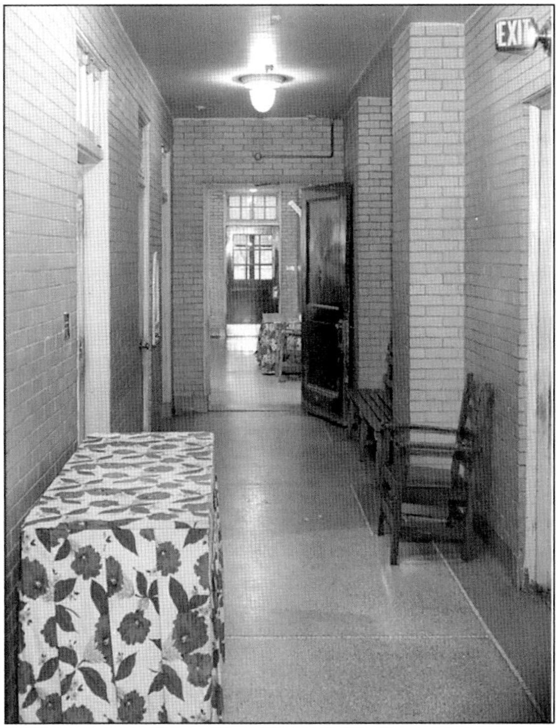

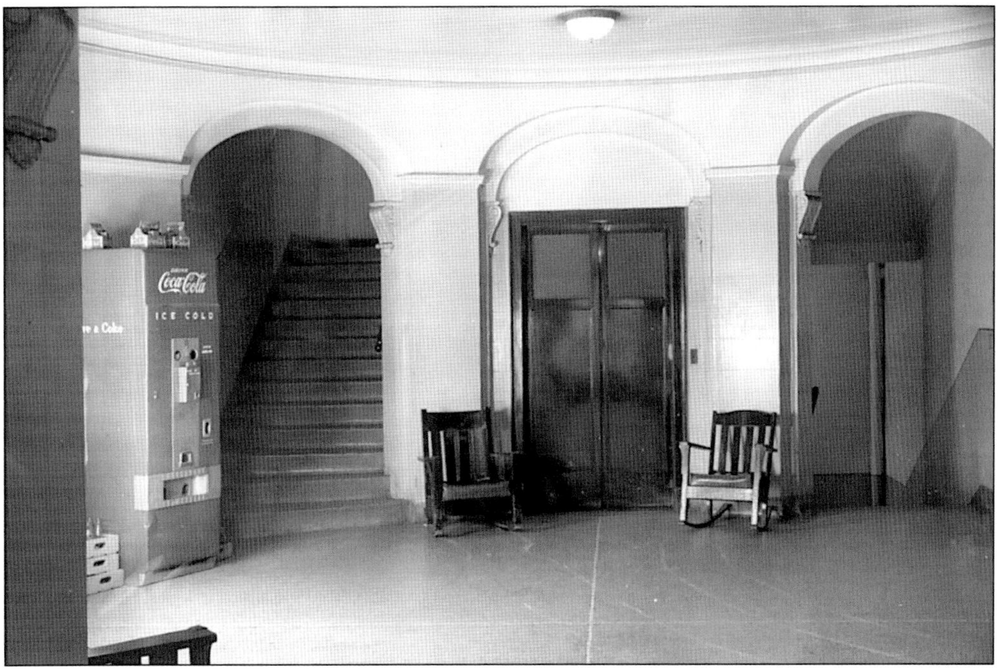

LOBBY OF "J" BUILDING, c. 1940S. Visitors could quench their thirst with an ice cold bottle of Coca-Cola bought from the vending machine in the lobby of this building, which housed 374 female psychiatric patients. The building was vacated in 1973 and was used as the Wayne County Office on Aging for a while before it was torn down. (Courtesy Eloise Museum, Westland, Michigan.)

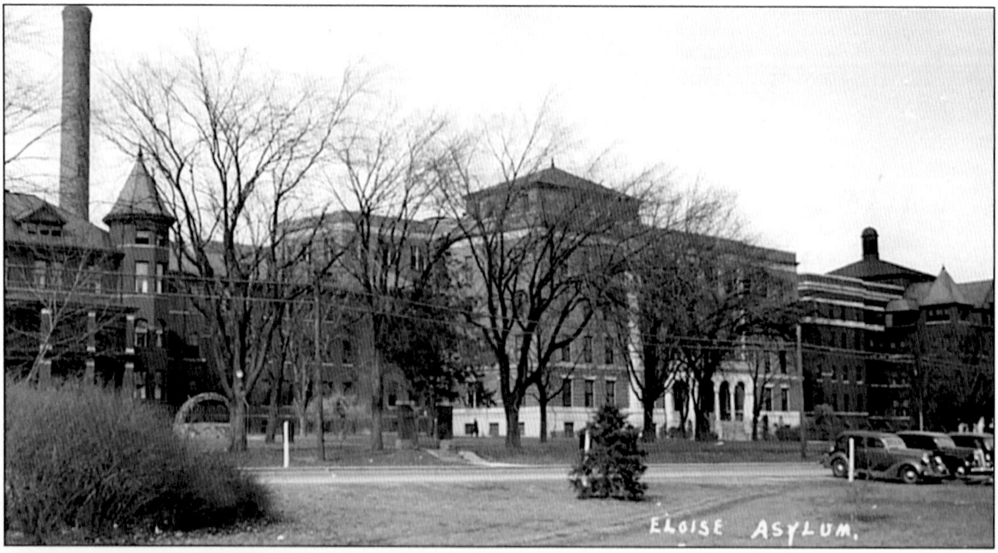

ELOISE ASYLUM, 1940S. This rare black and white postcard shows, from left to right, the asylum building, the administration building (D Building), and the William Seymour Hospital. Note the stone floral basket in front of the asylum building. The building is gone, but the basket is still there. Someone wrote on the front of this card "Where Sarah works." (Courtesy Eloise Museum, Westland, Michigan.)

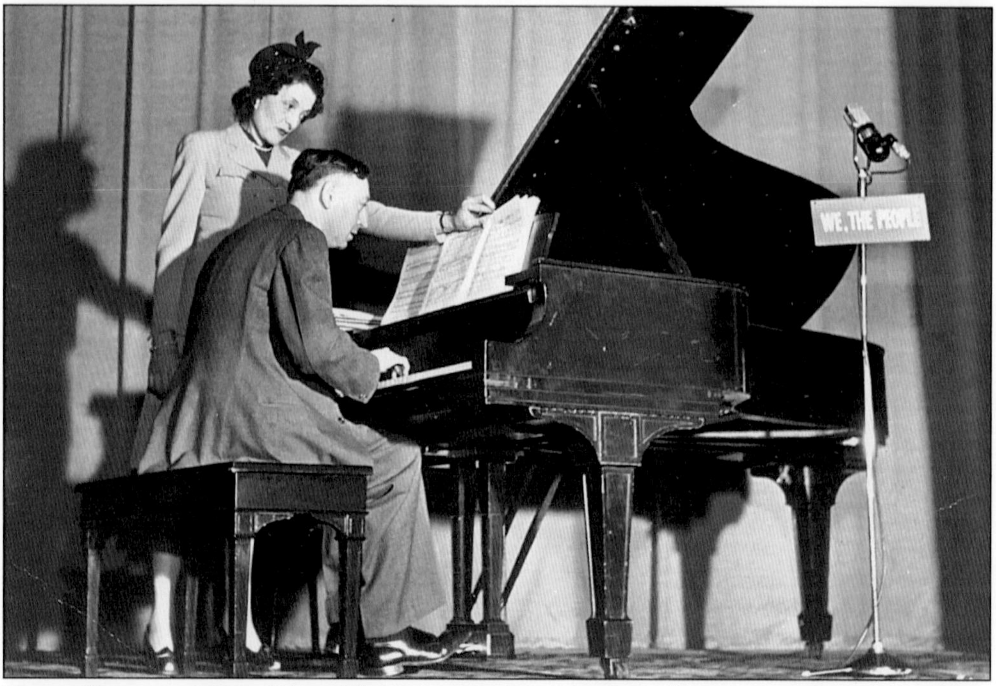

PIANO RECITAL, 1940S. Music Therapist Jane Matney turns the pages to the music while a patient gives a performance in the Gruber Auditorium. The pianist may be the famous "Dr. X," a psychiatric patient who was a professional musician whose concerts were broadcast twice on national radio. The first formal program in music therapy for mental patients was initiated at Eloise in 1937. (Courtesy Eloise Museum, Westland, Michigan.)

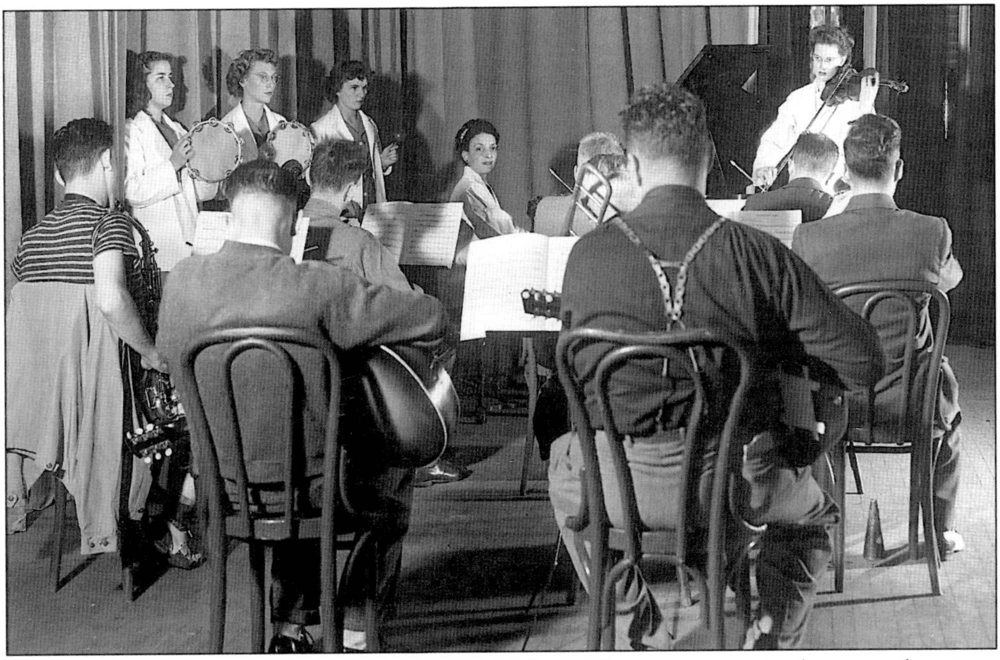

MORE MUSIC THERAPY, 1950S. Jane Matney, Music Therapist, is again shown at the piano with the Eloise music therapy orchestra. Staff members and music therapy interns (wearing lab coats) supplemented the patient musicians. (Courtesy Eloise Museum, Westland, Michigan.)

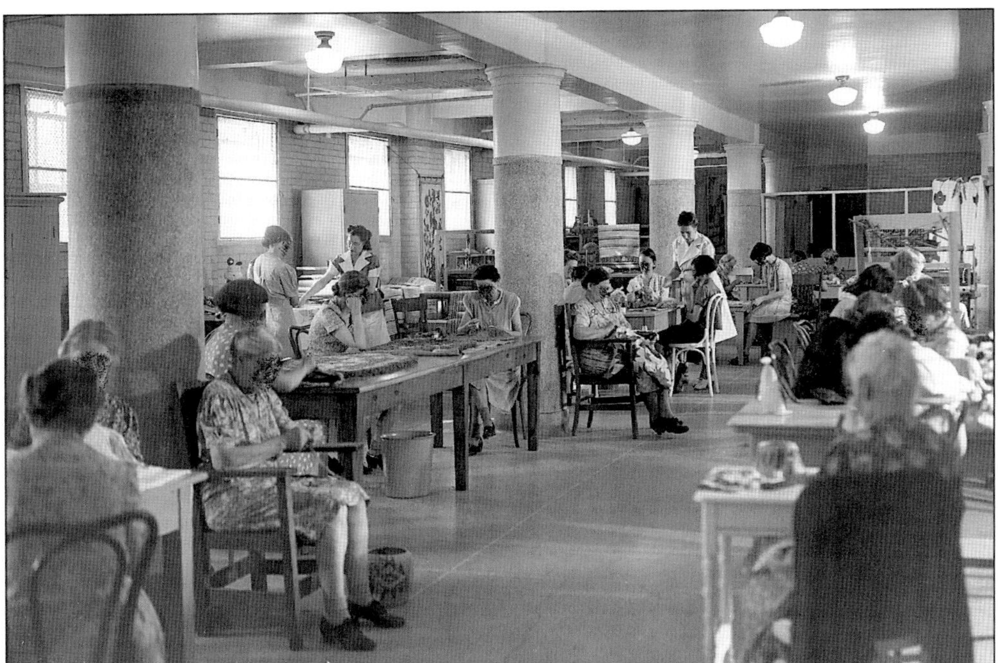

WOMEN'S OCCUPATIONAL THERAPY, 1950S. Staff and volunteers work with the mostly elderly psychiatric patients in the occupational therapy department. This photo was altered at the time it was taken so that patients could not be identified. (Courtesy Eloise Museum, Westland, Michigan.)

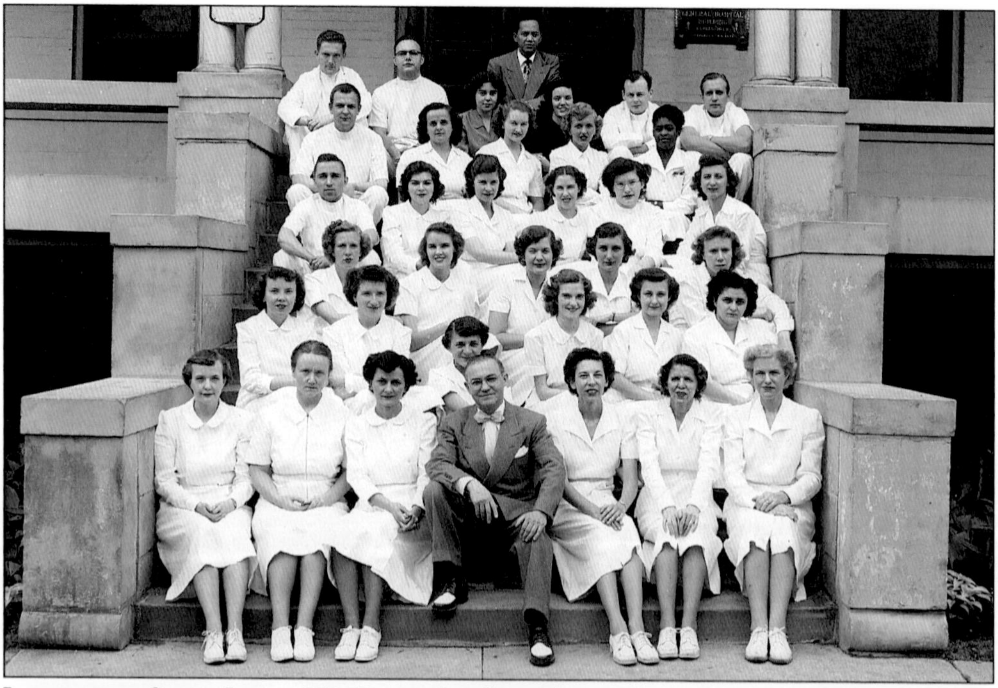

LABORATORY STAFF, JUNE 1950. Pictured staff members include, from left to right: (front row) B. Whitehouse, E. F.Leiser, A. Serafini, Sylvester E. Gould, R. Mason, G. Kercher, and E. Keay; (second row) S. Brewis, B. Levin, A. Johnson, M. Kingsbury, M. Ranson, and I. Block; (third row) P. Lessens, R. Homic, V. Bodick, M. Anderson, and P. Dietrich; (fourth row) R. Hines, B. Tuttle, L. Ripley, P. Kice, M. Buckley, and V. Stevens; (fifth row) D. White, E. Pelak, B. Toles, D. Moniuszko, and L. Dailey; (sixth row) L. Rose, L. Walter, R. Stempel, N. Rose, R. Ormond, and D. Van Hoek; and (seventh row) J. Arcellana. (Courtesy Westland Historical Museum.)

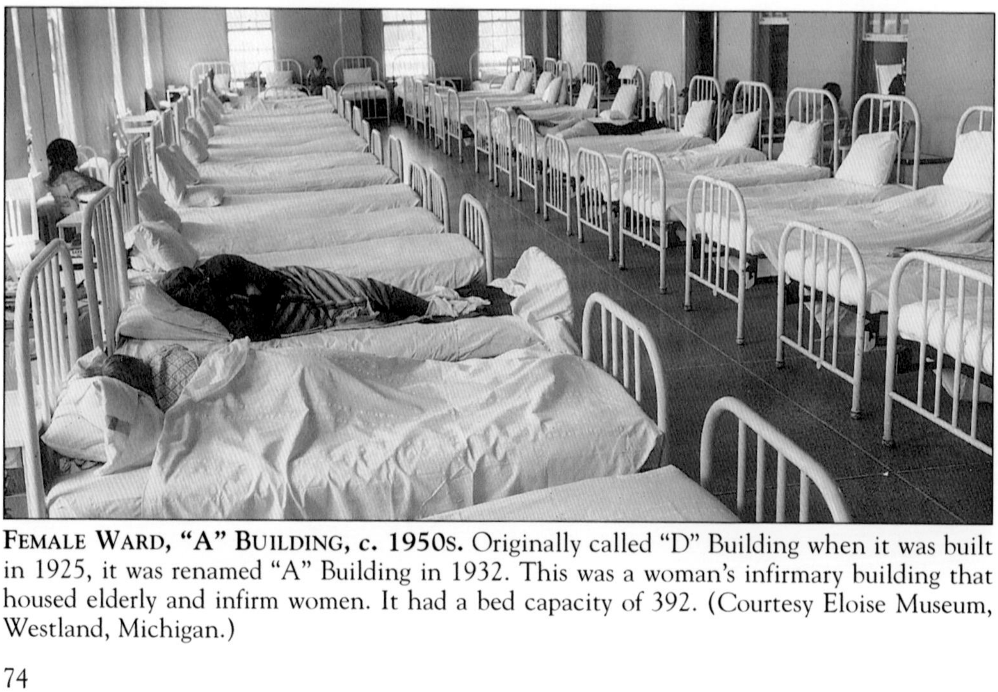

FEMALE WARD, "A" BUILDING, c. 1950S. Originally called "D" Building when it was built in 1925, it was renamed "A" Building in 1932. This was a woman's infirmary building that housed elderly and infirm women. It had a bed capacity of 392. (Courtesy Eloise Museum, Westland, Michigan.)

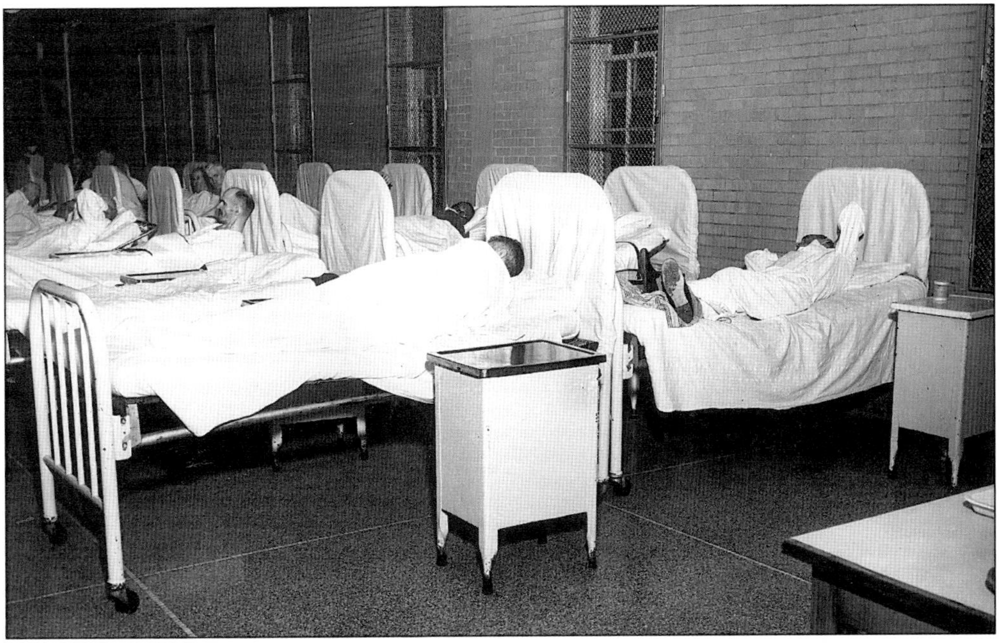

Male Psychiatric Ward, c. 1950s. This unidentified photo probably depicts the "M" Building, which for a time housed psychiatric patients who also had tuberculosis. Many of these men were alcoholics. "M" Building was put up in 1929 and was the last of the big psychiatric buildings. It was used as a Wayne County jail annex for a short time before it was torn down. (Courtesy Eloise Museum, Westland, Michigan.)

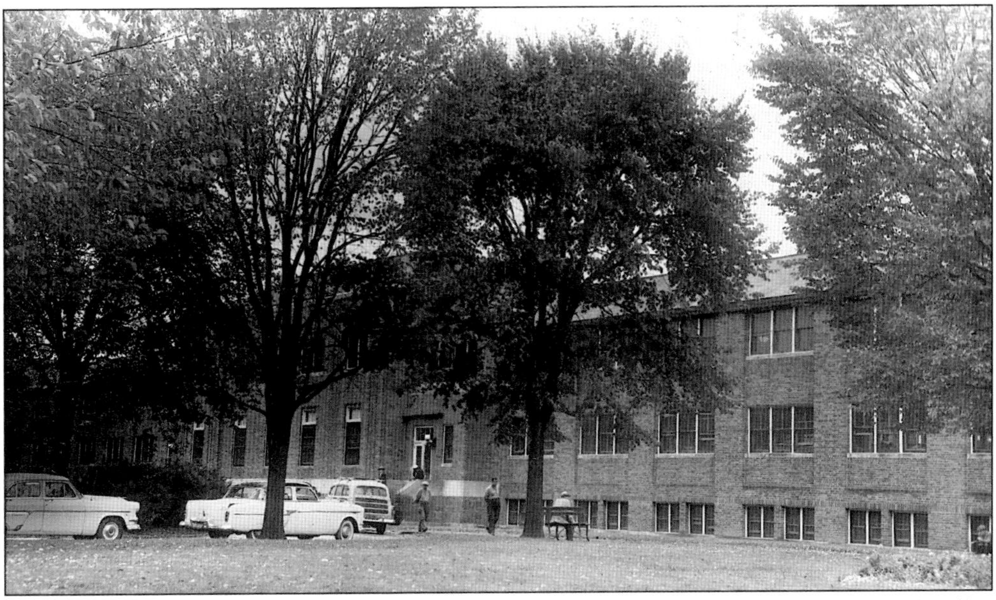

Kelley Hall or "N" Building, 1950s. A resident is sitting on a bench outside of Kelley Hall which was named for Frank E. Kelley who died June 18, 1954. Mr. Kelley was a life-long Detroit resident, a native of Old Corktown, and chairman of the Wayne County Board of County Institutions since 1943. Only a small portion of the enormous building that housed over 7,000 people is shown in this photo. (Courtesy Eloise Museum, Westland, Michigan.)

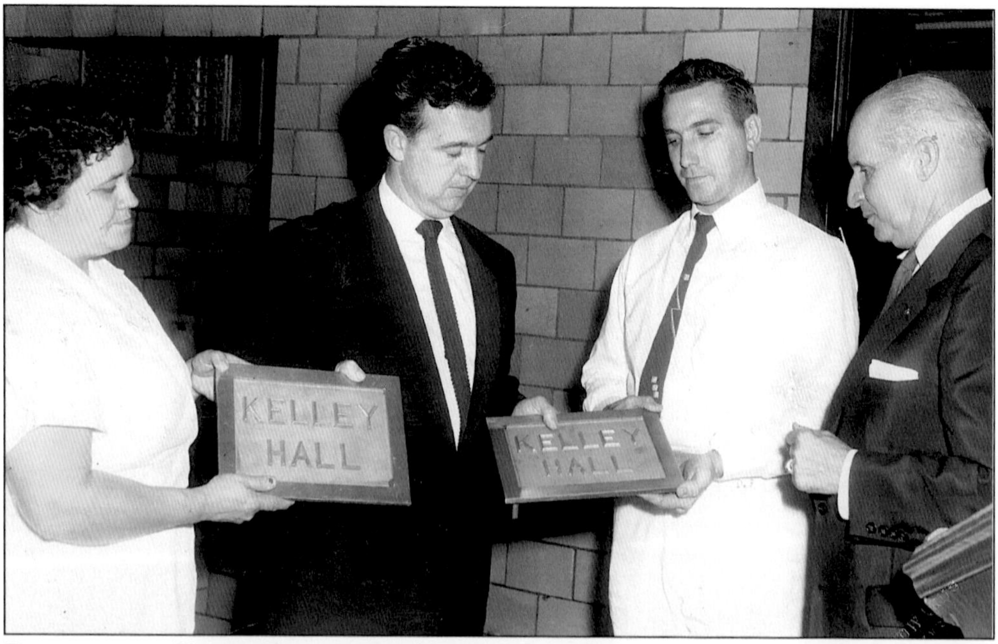

DEDICATION OF KELLEY HALL, 1950S. Two plaques with the name "Kelley Hall" are presented to employees by Frank Kelley Jr. and the mayor of Ecorse, William W. Voisine. Frank Kelley Jr. was the nation's longest-serving state Attorney General, serving in Michigan from 1961 until 1998. (Courtesy Eloise Museum, Westland, Michigan.)

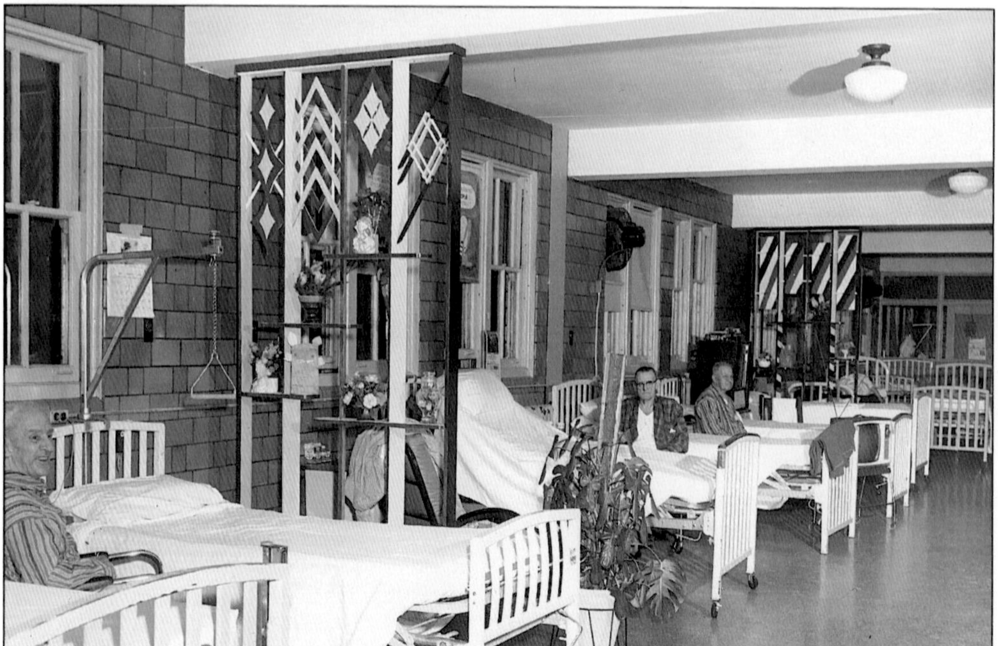

PATIENT WARD, KELLEY HALL, 1960S. Kelley Hall was used for chronically ill patients who spent months or even years there. Homey touches were added to the large wards to make them seem less institutional and more like home. (Courtesy Eloise Museum, Westland, Michigan.)

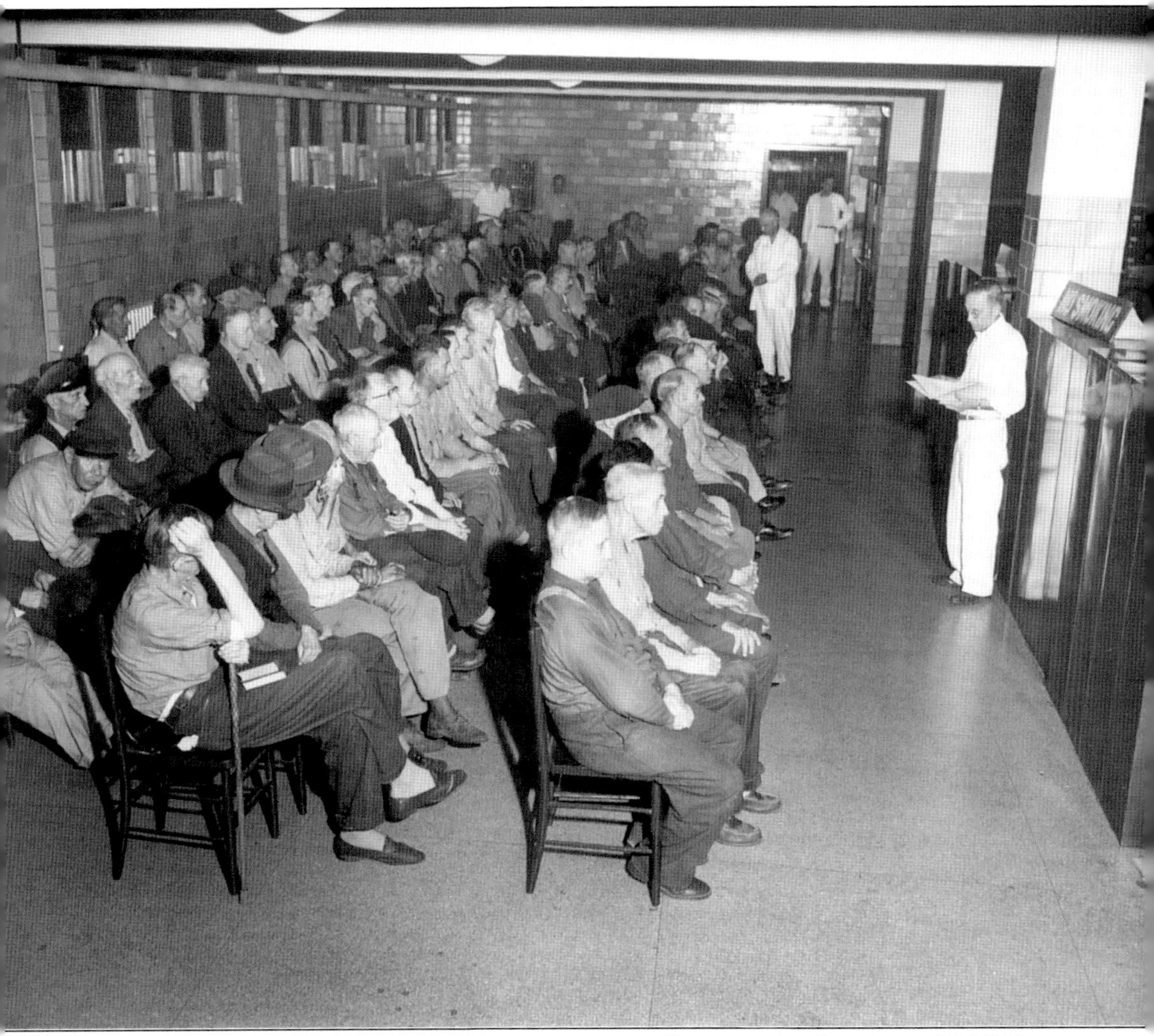

POGIES, KELLEY HALL, 1950S. These gentlemen were affectionately referred to as POGIES or Poor Old Guys in Eloise. In those days, these men would have been called tramps or bums, and now they are called the homeless. They were given free room and board in "N" Building, and in the winter months their numbers swelled to the thousands. Here they are being given instructions or work assignments by one of the ward attendants. Those who were able to work were given assignments, usually in the kitchen or cafeteria. Those who accepted work assignments were given special privileges. Note the NO SMOKING sign. Even back then, smoking was allowed only in designated areas. (Courtesy Eloise Museum, Westland, Michigan.)

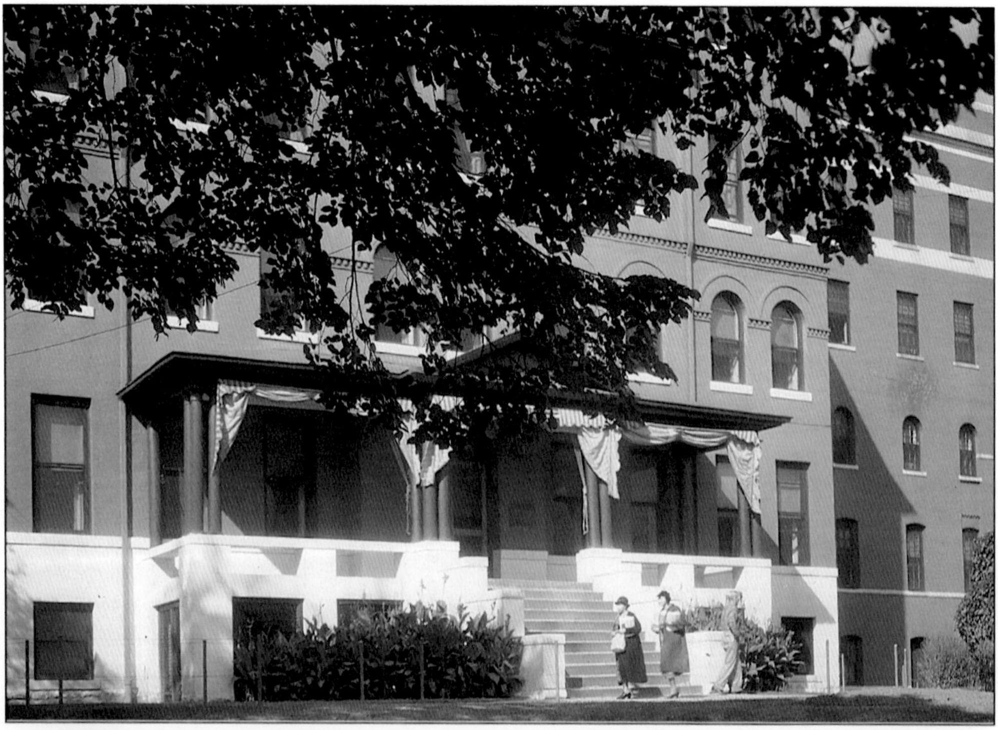

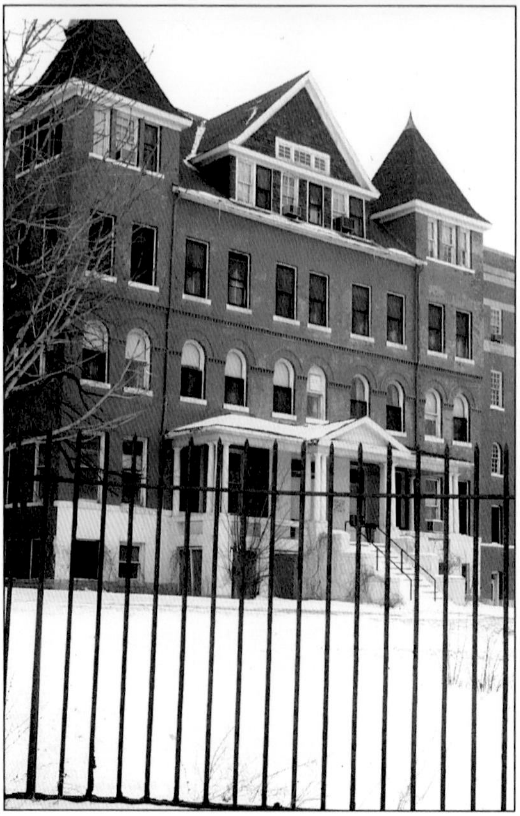

TWO VIEWS OF THE WILLIAM J. SEYMOUR HOSPITAL. This is the old Eloise Infirmary building remodeled into the first general hospital. Two ladies are walking in front the porch which is draped with bunting in the first photo, taken in the 1930s. The second photo was taken after the hospital closed, and the building was used for other purposes. (Courtesy Eloise Museum, Westland, Michigan.)

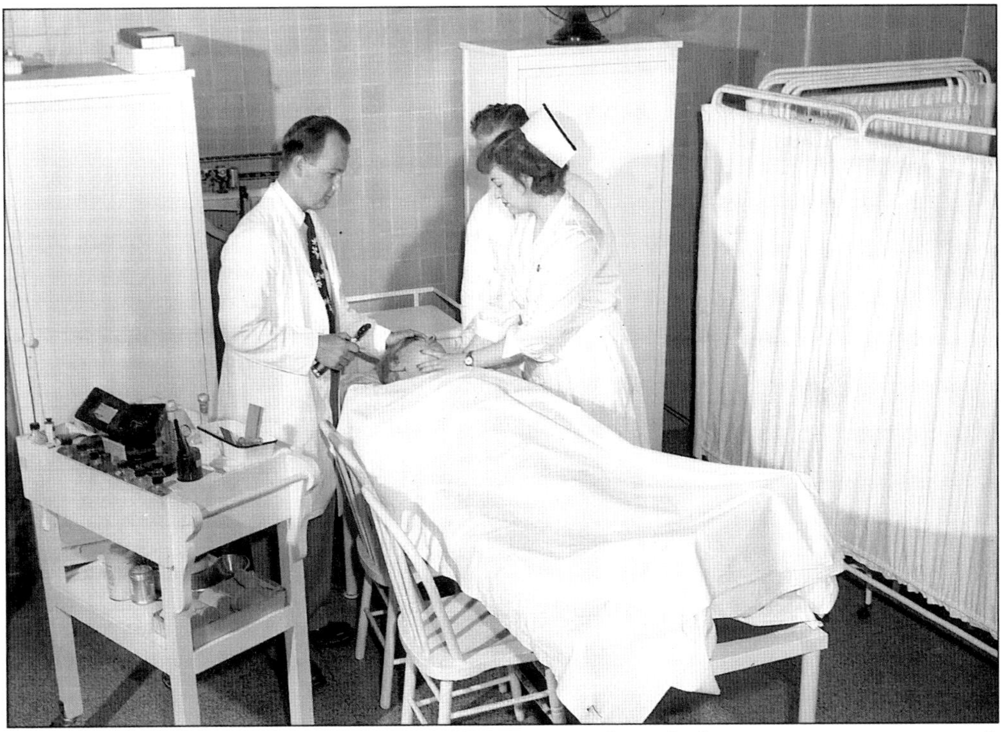

OUTPATIENT DEPARTMENT, SEYMOUR HOSPITAL, 1950S. A doctor examines a patient's retina while a nurse assists. (Courtesy Eloise Museum, Westland, Michigan.)

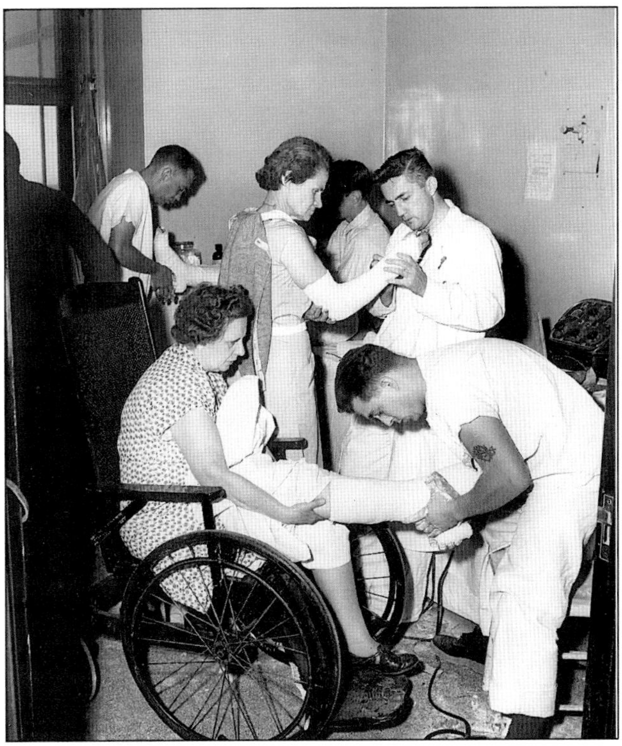

ORTHOPEDIC CLINIC, SEYMOUR HOSPITAL, 1950S. Patients are lined up to have plaster casts applied to fractured arms and legs in the busy cast room. The doctor at the rear is Ray D. Gaines. (Courtesy Eloise Museum, Westland, Michigan.)

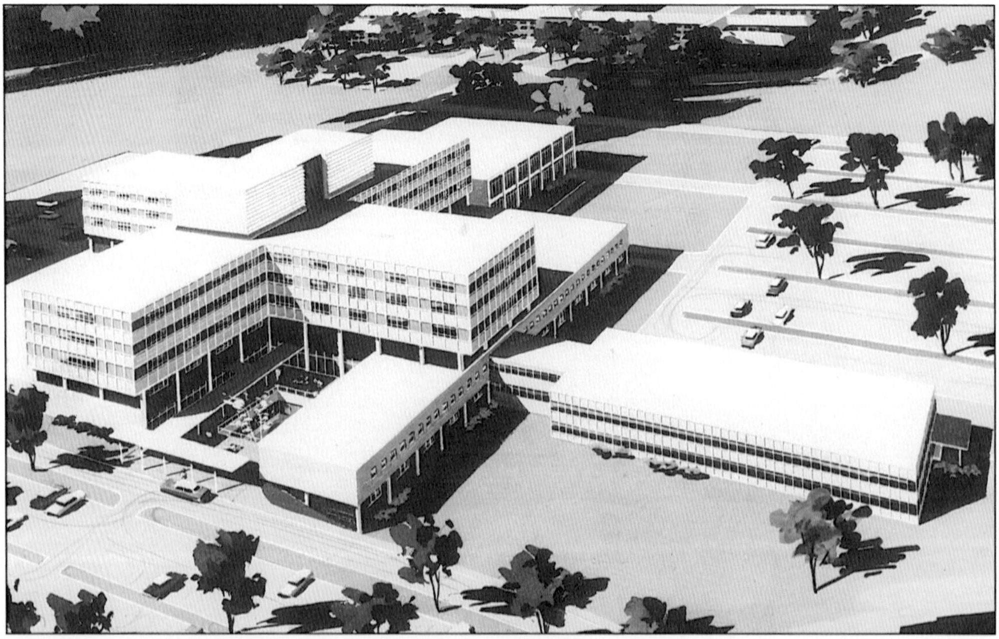

Proposed Model of New General Hospital, 1957. The architect's concept for the new hospital is shown in this model. The large building to the right is the hospital laundry which serviced all the buildings on the grounds. The large building to the rear of the hospital is "N" Building or Kelley Hall. (Courtesy Eloise Museum, Westland, Michigan.)

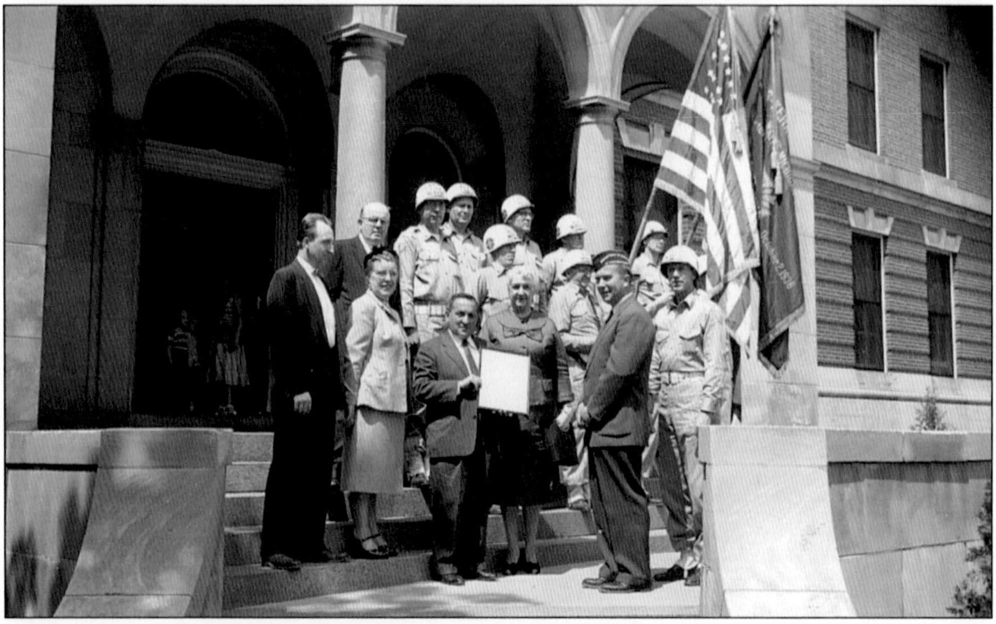

VFW Presentation on the Steps of "D" Building, 1956. Samuel Jacobson, the superintendent of Eloise, Martin Fleming, and Mrs. Margaret C. Doyle, members of the hospital board, are seen with the Harris-Kenren, VFW Wayne post. The marble staircase is no longer there, but "D" Building, now called the Kay Beard Building, is still being used for county offices today. (Courtesy Eloise Museum, Westland, Michigan.)

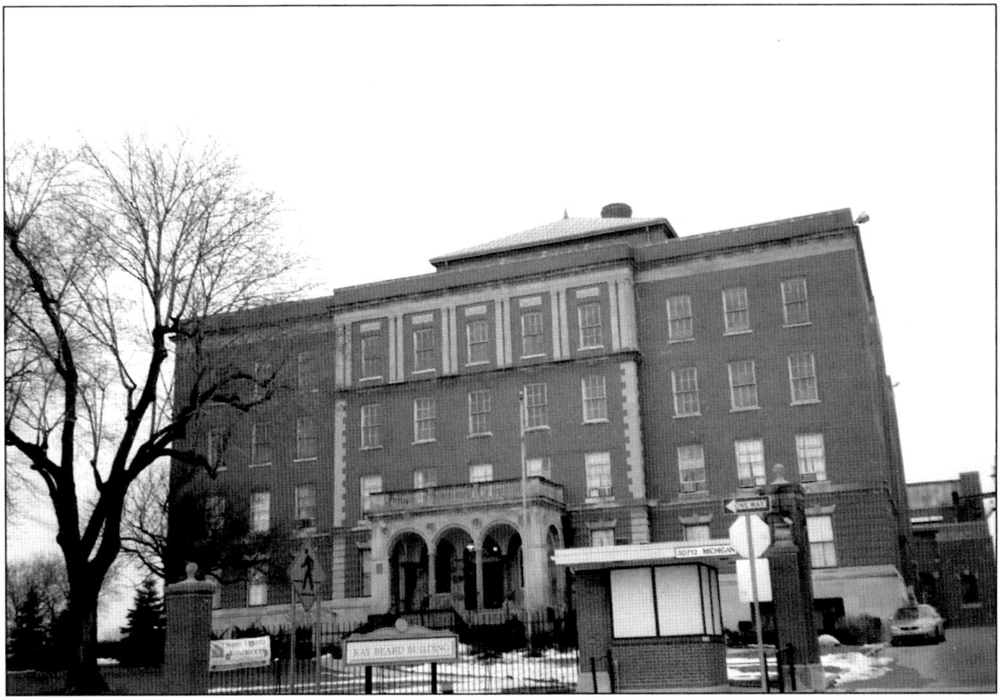

FRONT OF "D" BUILDING OR THE KAY BEARD BUILDING, 2002. This is how "D" building looks today. It was built in 1931 to house administrative offices, the post office, patient admission wards, and even had two complete apartments for employees on the third and fourth floors, as well as rooms for psychiatric attendants who lived on the grounds.

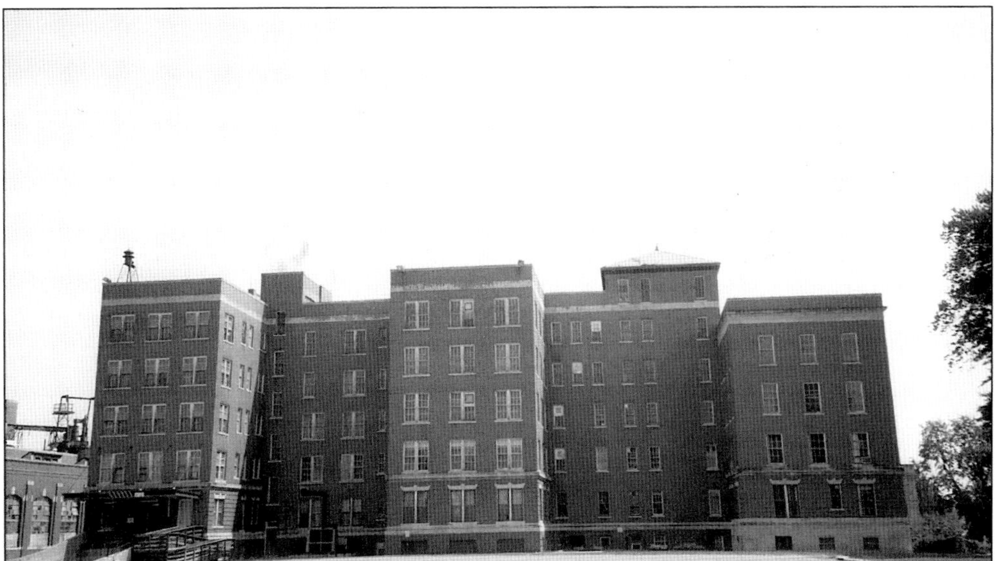

"D" BUILDING, 2002. This is a side view taken from the west side of the building which shows the loading dock. The size of the building can best be seen from this perspective. In addition to administrative offices and employee apartments, it housed 409 patients. In 1931, the year this structure was built, the total number of mental patients at Eloise was 3,488.

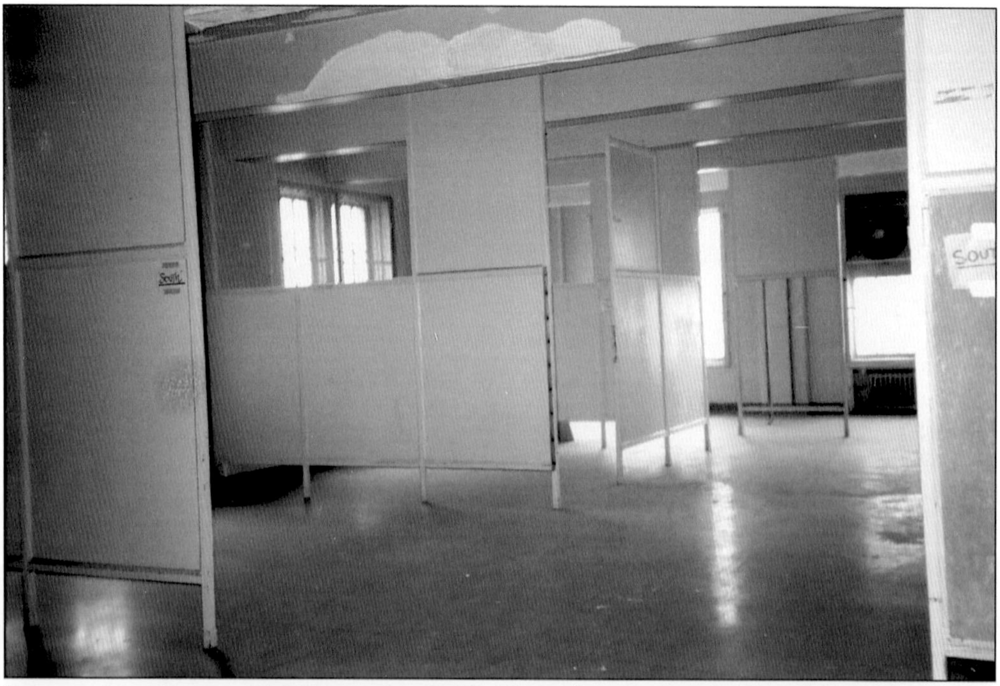

PSYCHIATRIC WARDS, "D" BUILDING, 2002. This is how the psychiatric wards looked at the time the hospital closed in 1977. The once-large open wards had been partitioned into smaller cubicles. These floors are currently vacant.

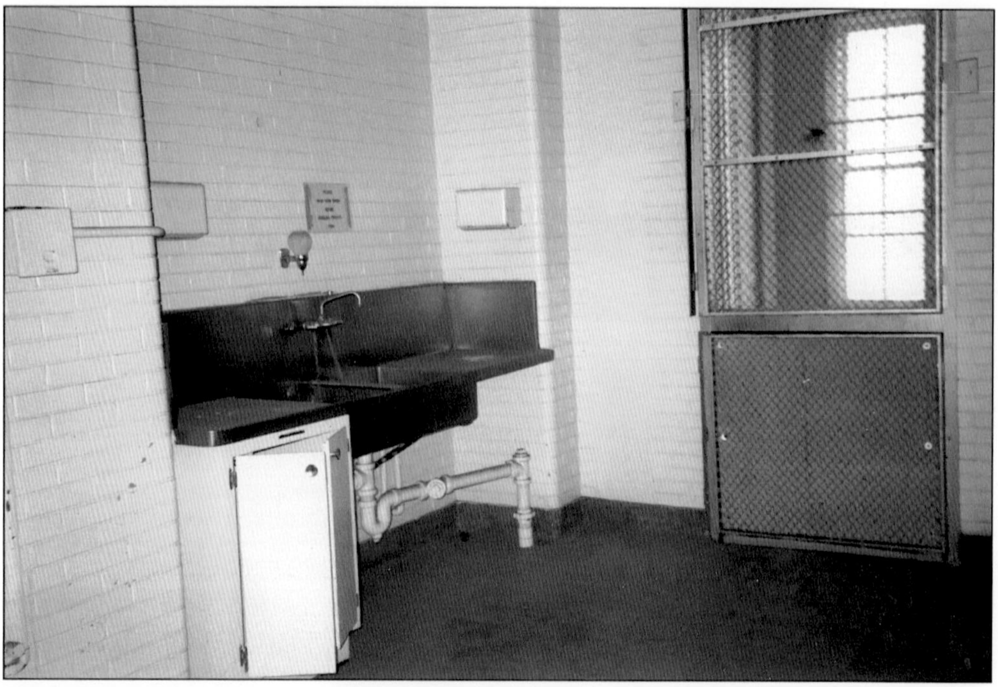

TREATMENT AREA, "D" BUILDING, 2002. This area is directly adjoining the sun porches which were on every floor.

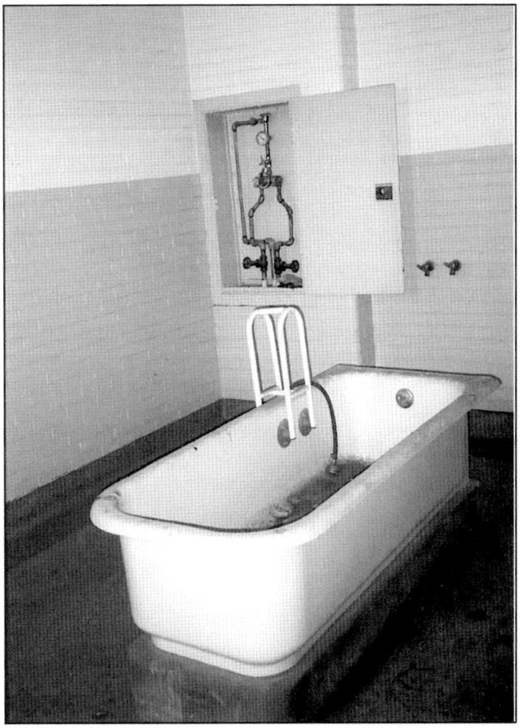

HYDROTHERAPY TUB, "D" BUILDING, 2002. Hydrotherapy was once used as a treatment to calm psychiatric patients. This tub hasn't been used in about 30 years, and this form of treatment for mental disorders is considered obsolete. Other early treatments were electroshock therapy, insulin therapy, music therapy, television therapy, and even malarial therapy.

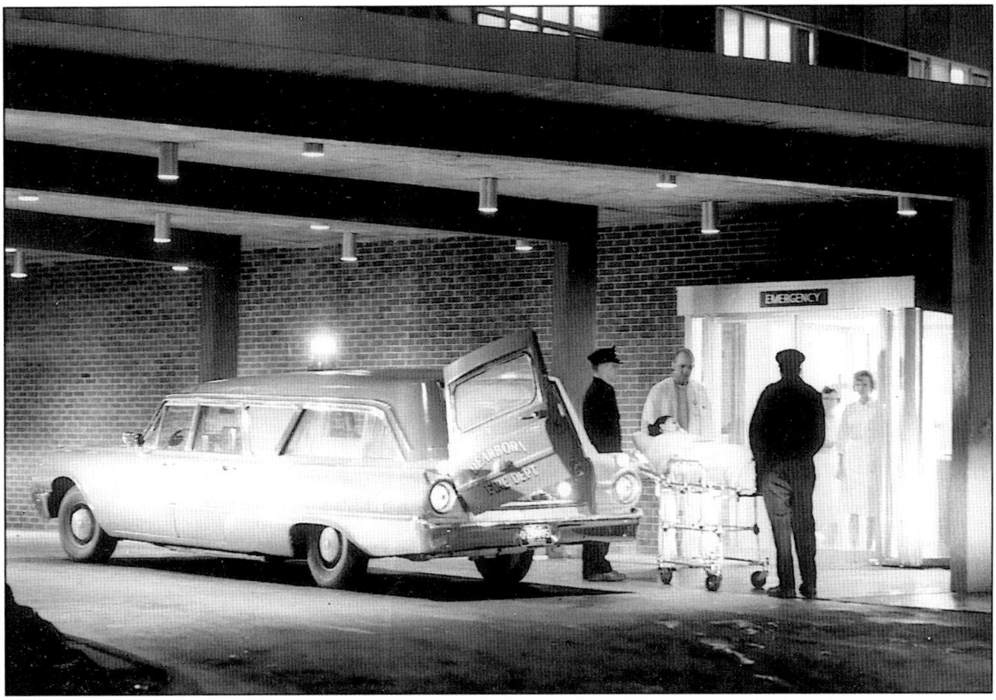

AMBULANCE ENTRANCE, WAYNE COUNTY GENERAL HOSPITAL, 1960S. Juanita Brannock, R.N., and Julie Vanger, R.N., both nursing supervisors, greet a patient brought to the hospital in a 1961 Ford ambulance by the Dearborn Fire Department. This was a very busy emergency room which was utilized by all communities in the area. (Courtesy Eloise Museum, Westland, Michigan.)

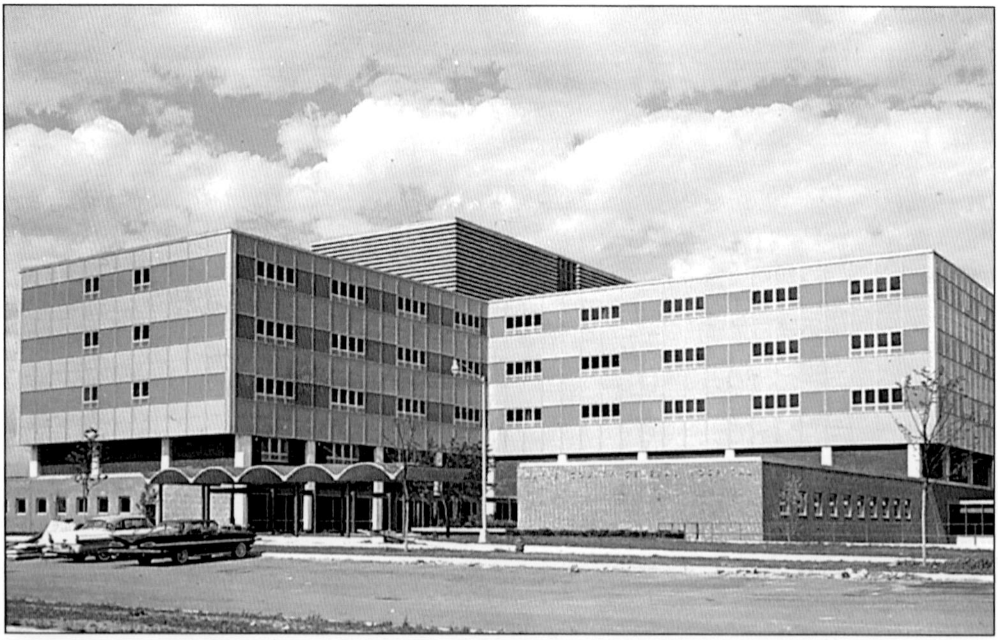

POSTCARD OF WAYNE COUNTY GENERAL HOSPITAL, 1970S. This building stood for only 38 years before it was razed. It was built in 1962 and razed in 2000. The 500-bed hospital was the only Level 1 trauma hospital for western Wayne County. It housed the first kidney dialysis unit in the state of Michigan. No patient was ever turned away because of lack of money or insurance. (Courtesy Eloise Museum, Westland, Michigan.)

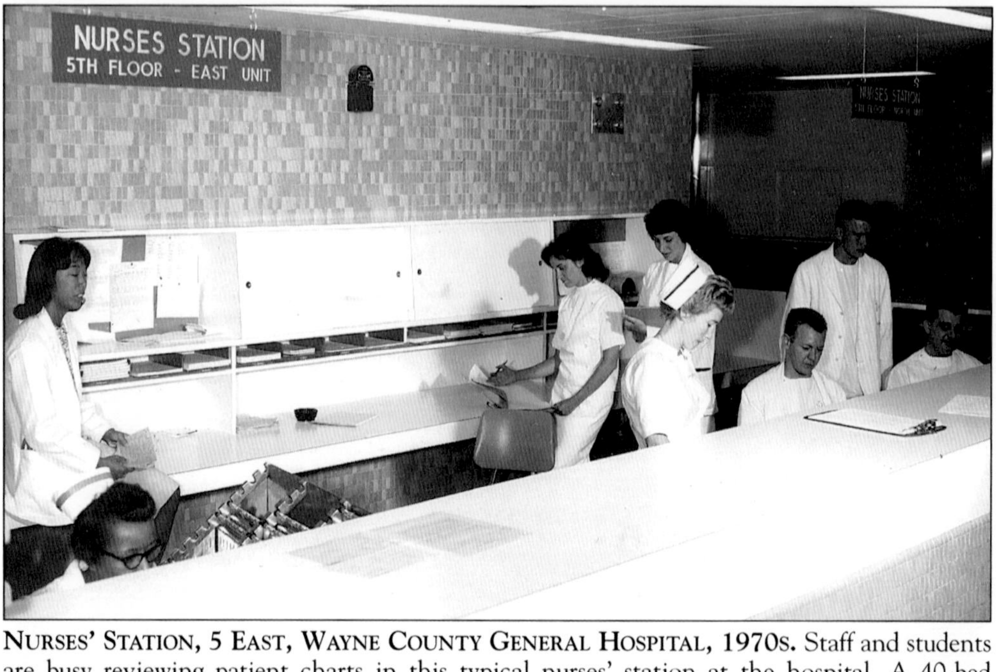

NURSES' STATION, 5 EAST, WAYNE COUNTY GENERAL HOSPITAL, 1970S. Staff and students are busy reviewing patient charts in this typical nurses' station at the hospital. A 40-bed medical unit, 5 East was also home to the home training kidney dialysis unit. (Courtesy Eloise Museum, Westland, Michigan.)

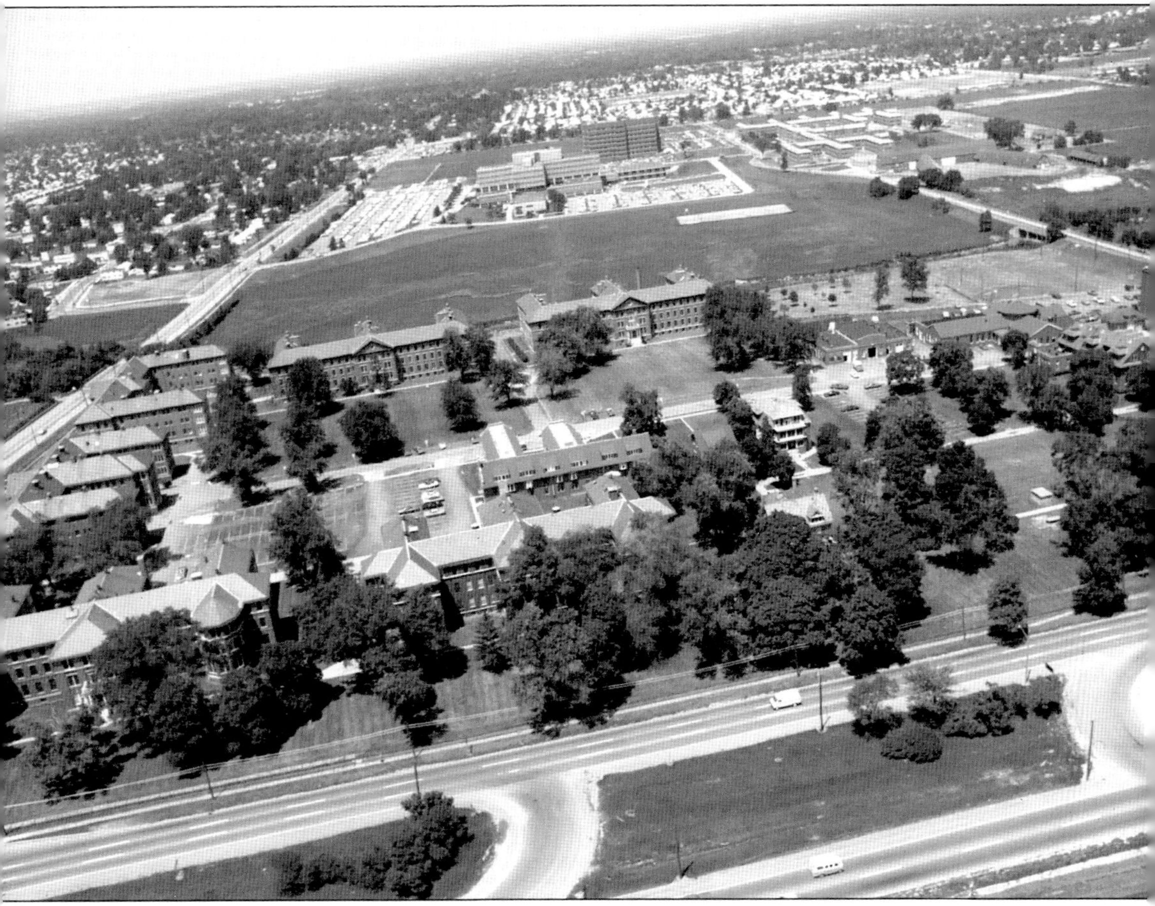

Aerial View of Eloise Psychiatric Complex, 1970s. This photo shows the large psychiatric buildings from the perspective of Michigan Avenue. At one time Wayne County cared for more mental patients here than all the state mental institutions combined. These buildings were closed in 1973 and the patients were transferred to state mental institutions. The general hospital, Walter P. Reuther Hospital, and "N" Building or Kelley Hall are in the background. At one time this complex stood on 902 acres of land, complete with about 70 buildings, of which only five are still standing. It was large enough to have its own post office, and mail from here was postmarked "Eloise, Michigan." (Courtesy Eloise Museum, Westland, Michigan.)

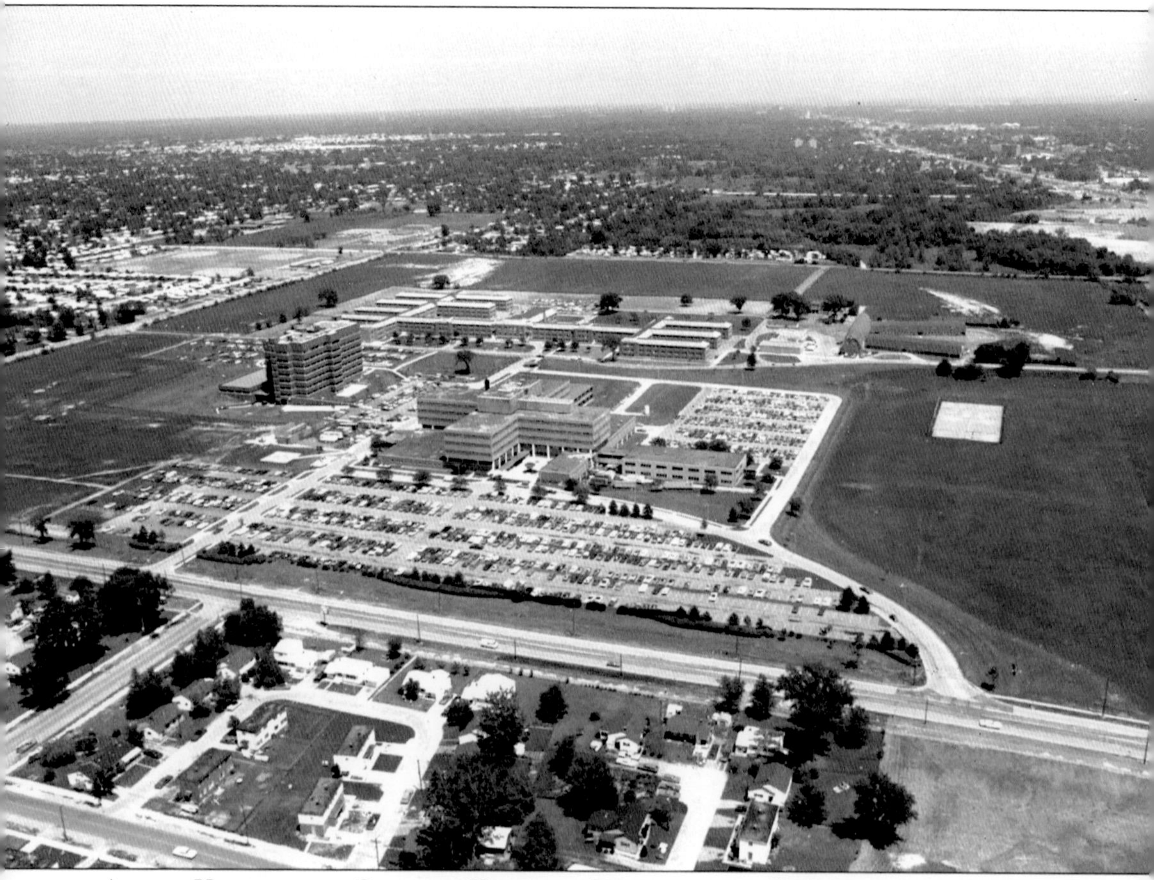

AERIAL VIEW OF THE GENERAL HOSPITAL, REUTHER AND "N" BUILDING, 1970S. This photo shows Wayne County General Hospital, the Walter P. Reuther Hospital, and "N" Building or Kelley Hall from the perspective of Merriman Road. The houses south of Merriman are part of the Norwayne project. Eloise was unique because Wayne County was the only one of Michigan's 83 counties that operated a psychiatric hospital, a general hospital, and an infirmary division all at the same place. (Courtesy Eloise Museum, Westland, Michigan.)

Four

THE VISITING NURSE ASSOCIATION OF DETROIT

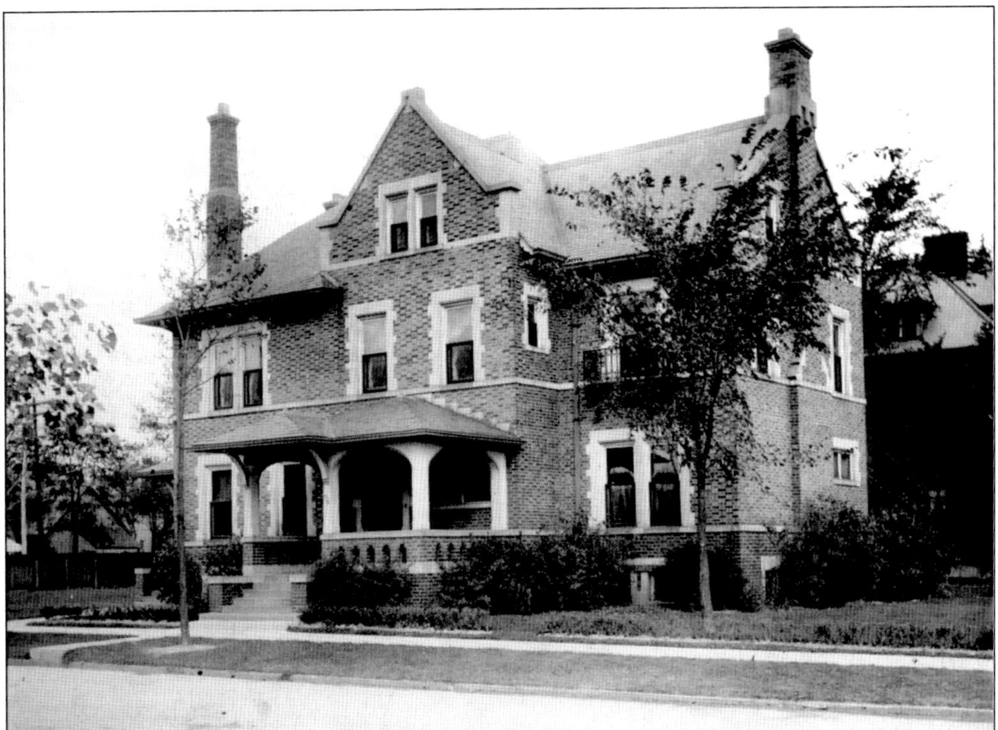

FIRST HEADQUARTERS OF THE VISITING NURSE ASSOCIATION. The VNA was founded in 1898. This house was donated by Mrs. Tracy McGregor and was located at the corner of Brush and Forest Streets in Detroit. The first tuberculosis clinic in Detroit was established in 1906 by the VNA in a partnership with the Detroit Board of Health. (Courtesy Burton Historical Collection, Detroit Public Library.)

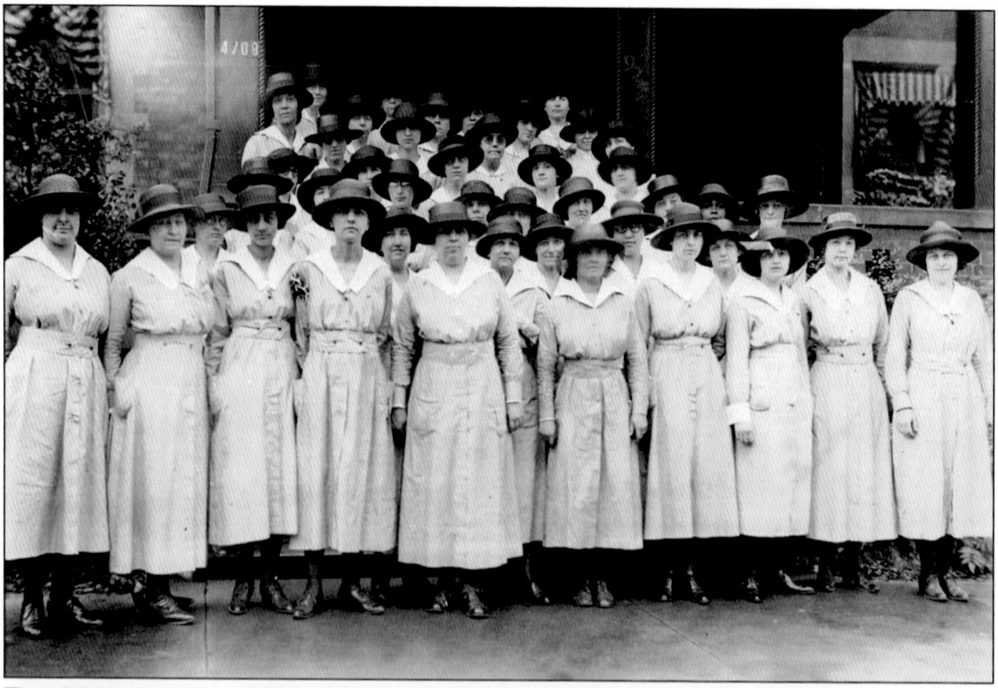

THE VNA STAFF, c. 1922. This group photo was taken in front of the first headquarters building. The windows were fitted up with awnings at the time the photo was taken. In 1911, the Metropolitan Life Insurance Company became the first to pay the VNA for home visits to industrial policy holders. (Courtesy Burton Historical Collection, Detroit Public Library.)

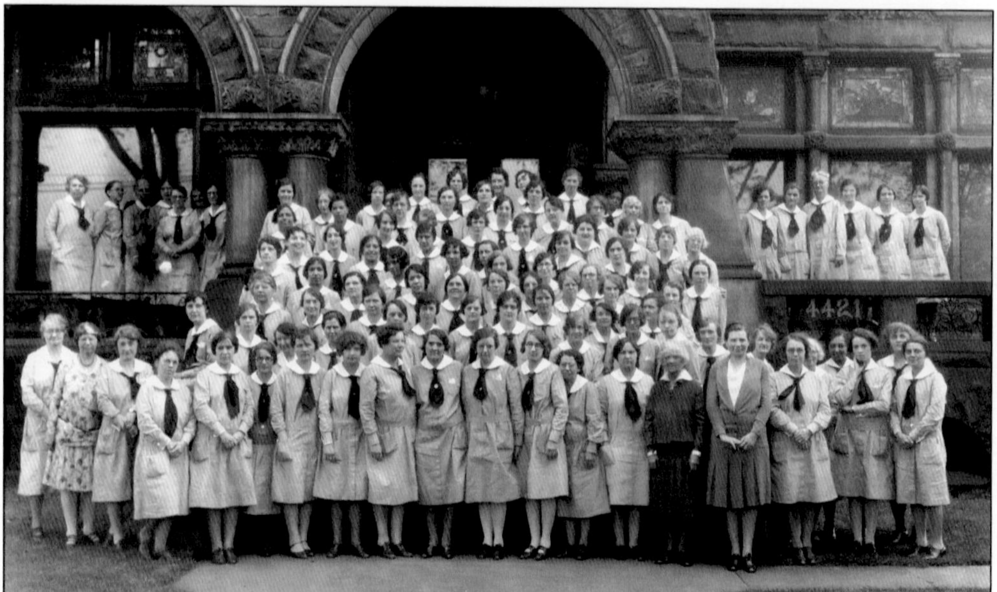

THE VNA STAFF, c. 1928. The entire staff is posed in front of their new headquarters with director Emilie Sargent and retired director Lystra Grettel. The VNA was in a partnership with the YMCA and the Urban League as members of the Detroit Patriotic Fund, a forerunner to the United Foundation. (Courtesy Burton Historical Collection, Detroit Public Library.)

THE VISITING NURSE, 1930S. This woman was one of a staff of 120 registered nurses who operated from 11 centers in Detroit, Michigan, and made over 200,000 home visits a year. In addition to nursing care, the association provided nutrition services, physiotherapy, occupational therapy, and healthy baby clinics. (Courtesy Burton Historical Collection, Detroit Public Library.)

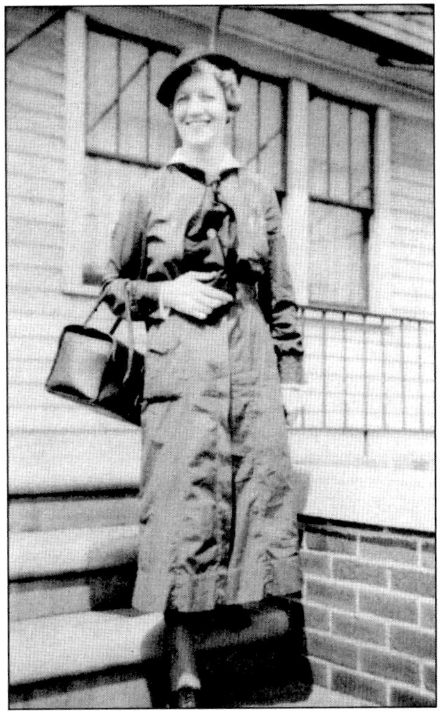

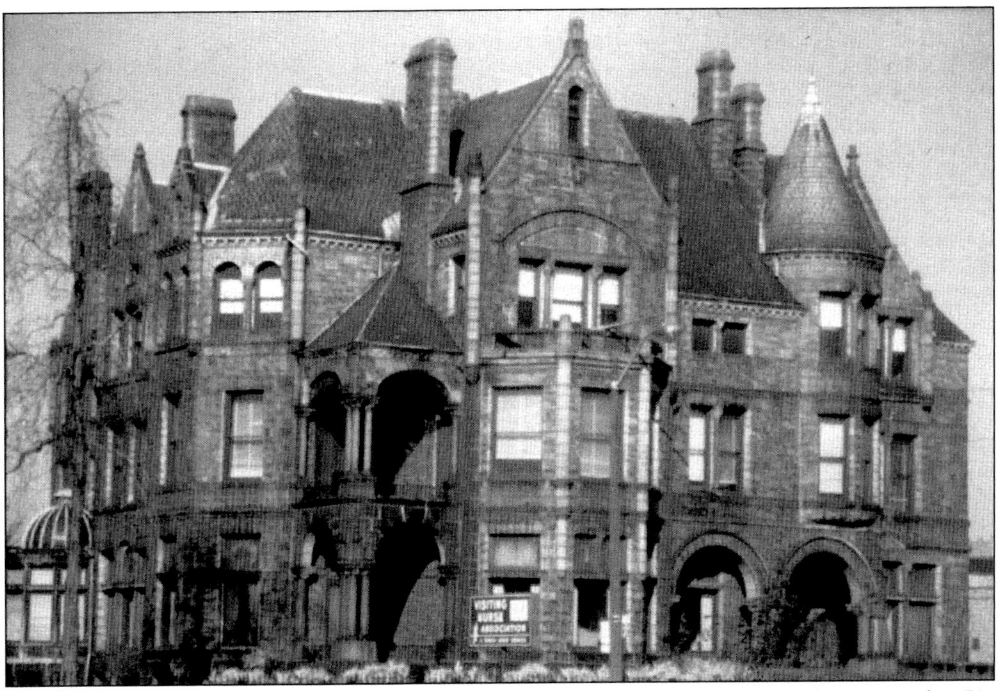

THE WHITNEY, c. 1950. Now a famous Detroit restaurant at 4421 Woodward Avenue, this 52-room mansion was built in 1894 by the lumber baron David Whitney Jr. He died in 1900, and the home was used by his family until about 1920. It was then the headquarters for the Wayne County Medical Society followed by the Visiting Nurse Association for many years. (Courtesy Burton Historical Collection, Detroit Public Library.)

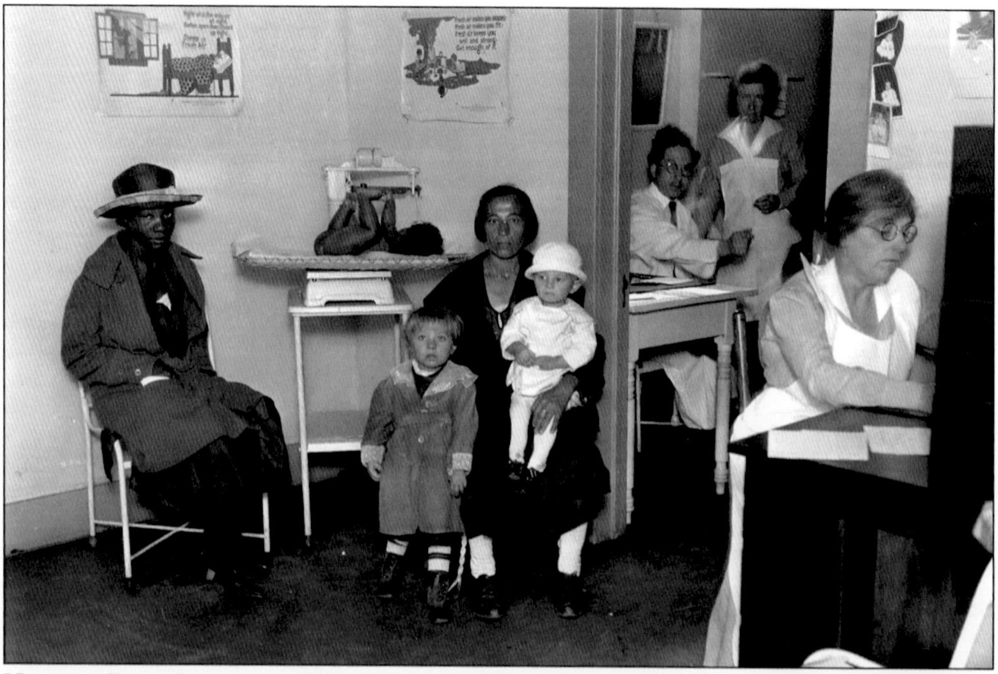

HEALTHY BABY CLINIC, c. 1920S. Here a cute baby on the scale is playing with his feet while his mother waits to talk to the visiting nurse. These clinics were first opened in 1914 to improve infant health during a time when there was a large influx of immigrants into Detroit. These clinics were free to those unable to pay. (Courtesy Burton Historical Collection, Detroit Public Library.)

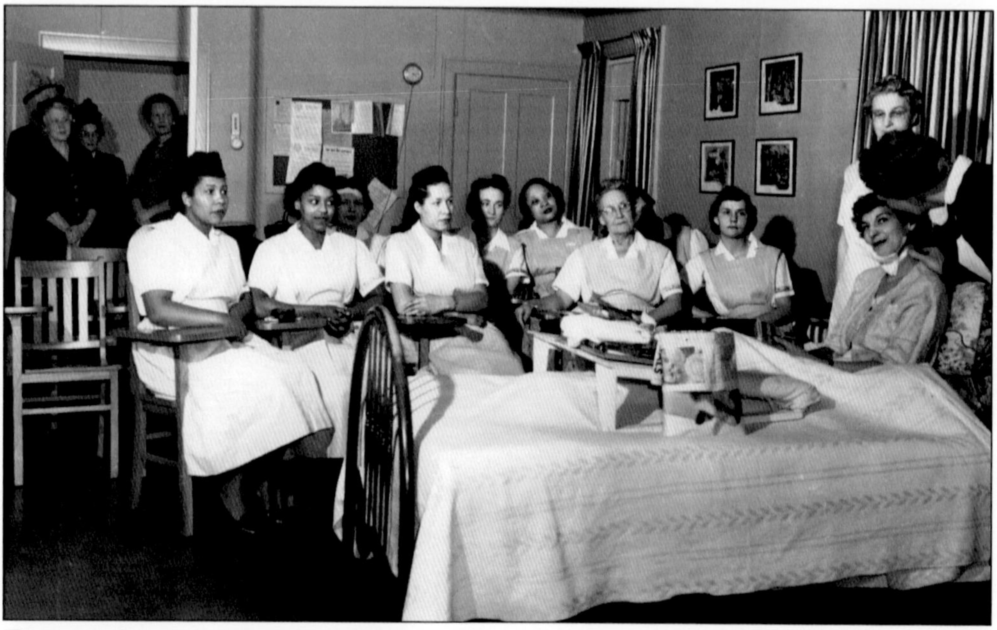

TRAINING SESSION, 1950S. Mrs. Carolyn Derrington, at far right bending over, is demonstrating how to care for a cancer patient in her home. The "patient" is Mrs. Victoria Schaedel, a student nurse. Members of the Board of Trustees are standing in the doorway. (Courtesy Burton Historical Collection, Detroit Public Library.)

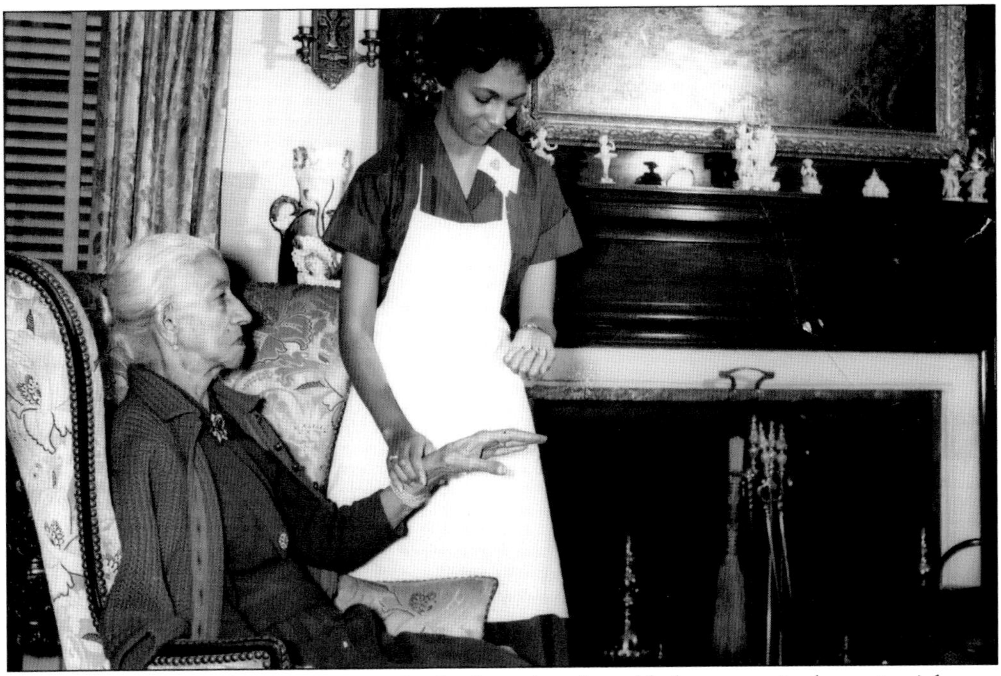

CHECKING A PULSE. A visiting nurse checks the pulse of an elderly woman in the patient's home. These home visits increased both the comfort and independence of the patient. By 1959, the VNA had extended service to Oakland County. It is now known as the Visiting Nurse Association of Southeast Michigan. (Courtesy Burton Historical Collection, Detroit Public Library.)

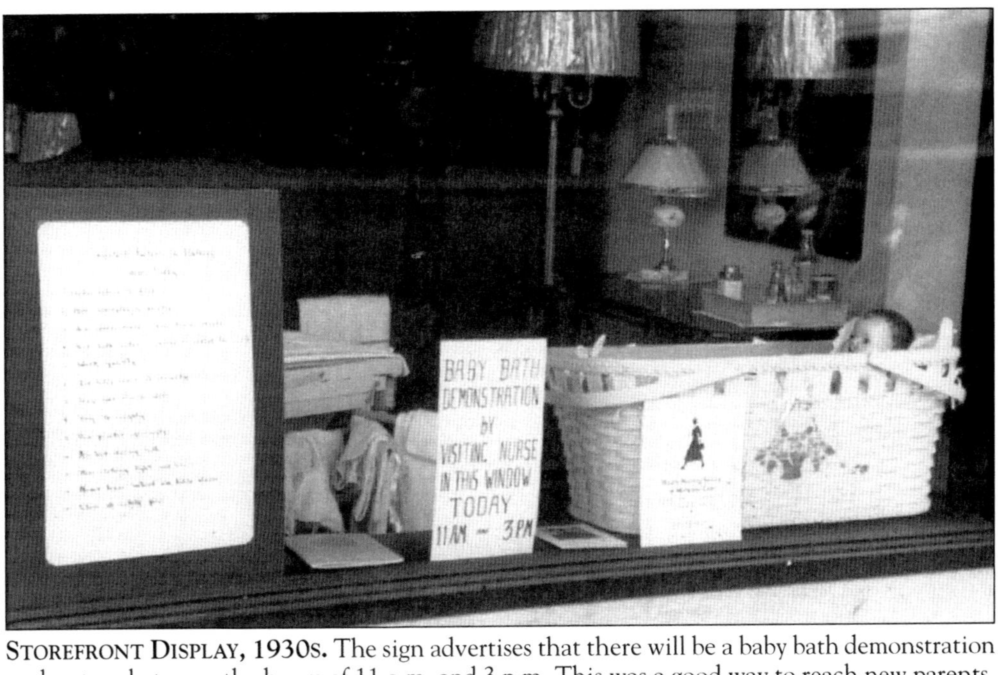
BABY BATH
DEMONSTRATION
BY
VISITING NURSE
IN THIS WINDOW
TODAY
11AM - 3PM

STOREFRONT DISPLAY, 1930S. The sign advertises that there will be a baby bath demonstration at the store between the hours of 11 a.m. and 3 p.m. This was a good way to reach new parents. In the 1960s the VNA established the Mom and Tots Family Center. (Courtesy Burton Historical Collection, Detroit Public Library.)

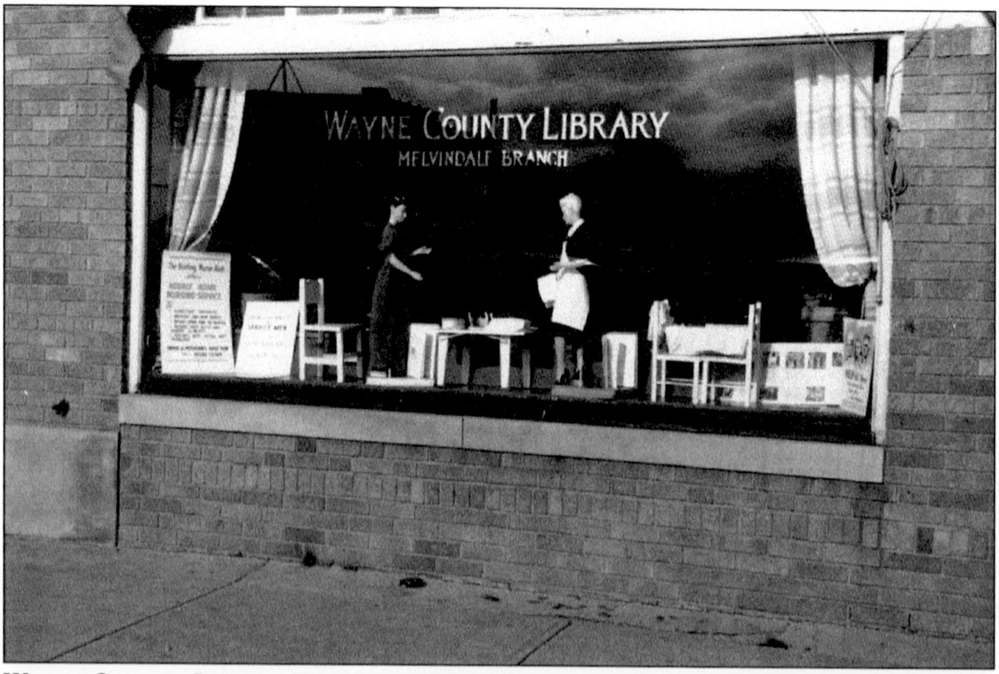

WAYNE COUNTY LIBRARY DISPLAY, 1930S. The front window of the Melvindale Branch of the Wayne County Library is a showcase for services provided at the time by the Visiting Nurse Association. (Courtesy Burton Historical Collection, Detroit Public Library.)

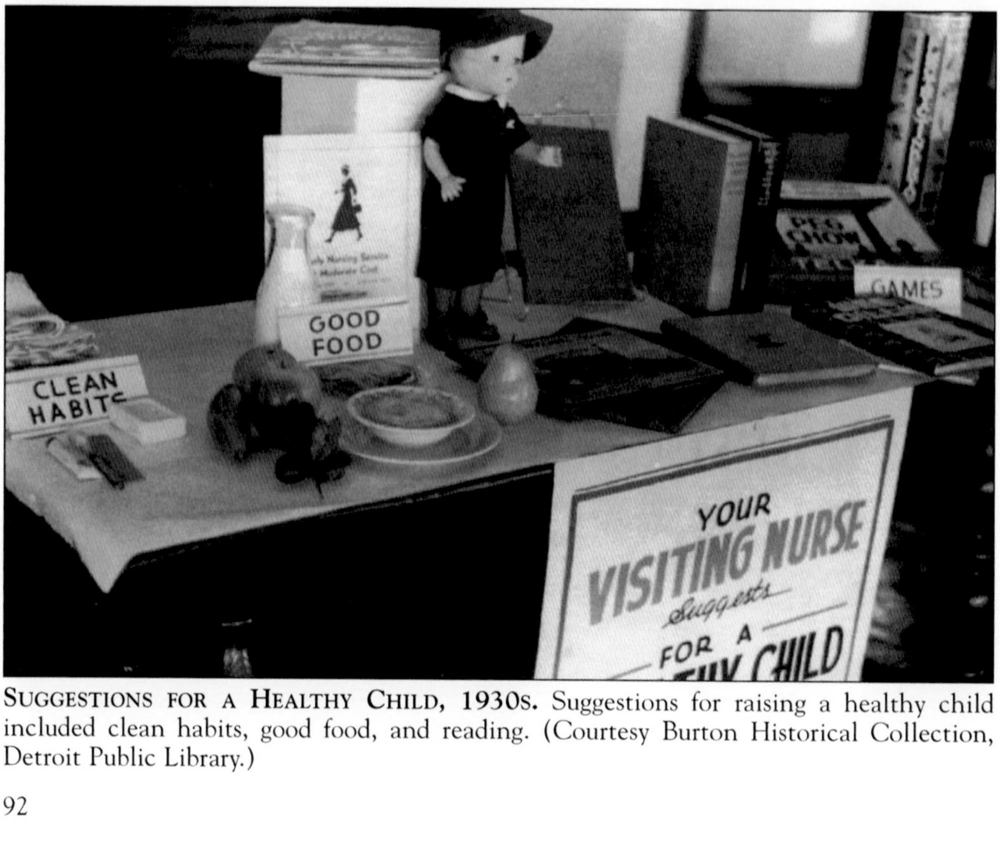

SUGGESTIONS FOR A HEALTHY CHILD, 1930S. Suggestions for raising a healthy child included clean habits, good food, and reading. (Courtesy Burton Historical Collection, Detroit Public Library.)

Five

Benevolent Societies

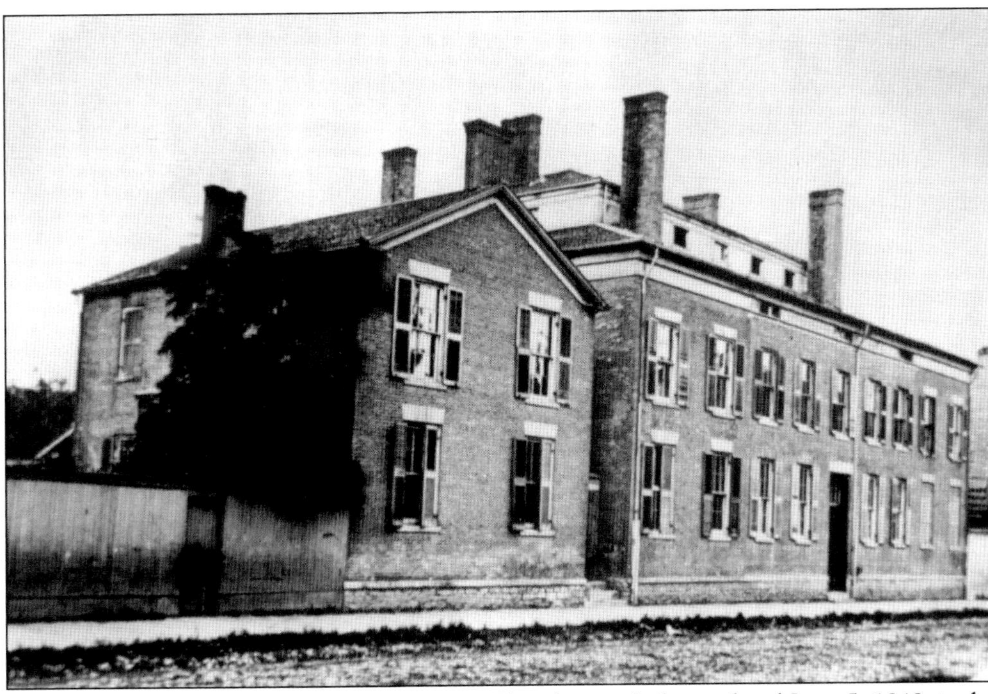

St. Vincent's Orphan Asylum, c. 1848. This damaged photo, dated June 5, 1848, is the only known photo of this early Detroit orphanage which was located at the corner of Randolph and Larned. The orphanage evolved from the Catholic Female Association which was organized in 1834 for the relief of the sick and poor in Detroit. (Courtesy Daughters of Charity Archives, Mater Dei Provincialate, Evansville, Indiana.)

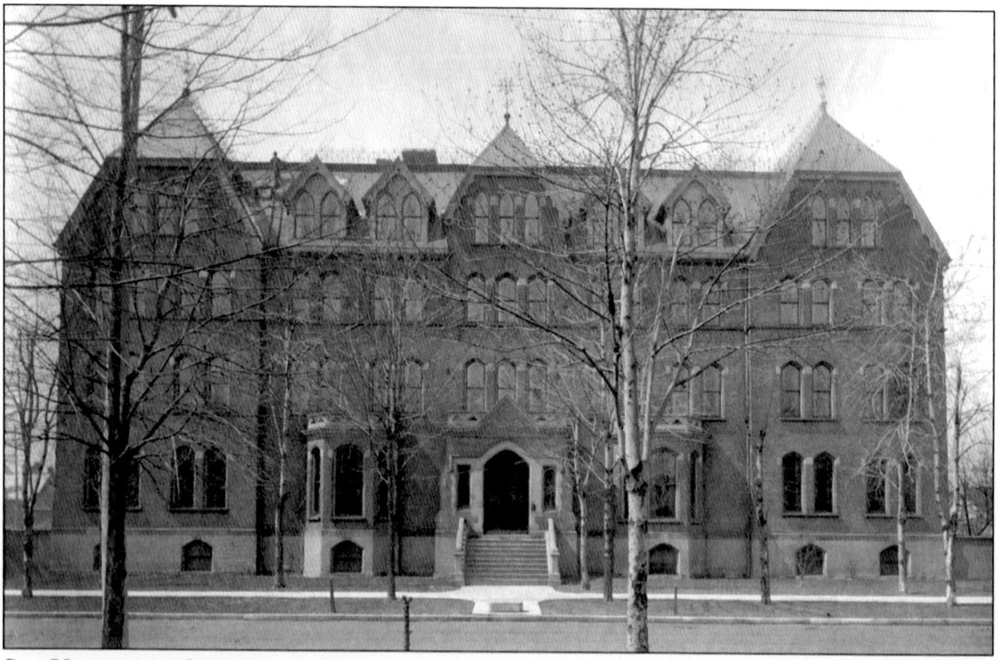

ST. VINCENT'S ORPHAN ASYLUM, c. 1876. This is a new orphanage building which was dependent upon voluntary contributions and the proceeds of an annual fair to care for the children. Up to 250 girls, aged two to twelve, were accommodated here. The sisters who were in charge were Sisters Loyola, Lucretia, Edmond, and Mary Stella. (Courtesy Daughters of Charity Archives, Mater Dei Provincialate, Evansville, Indiana.)

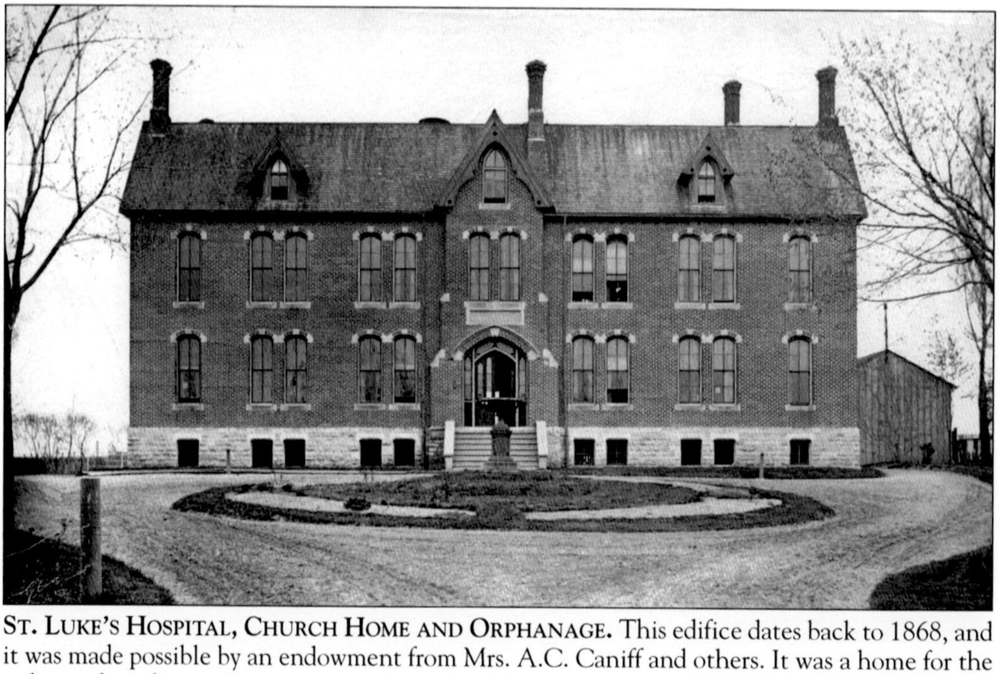

ST. LUKE'S HOSPITAL, CHURCH HOME AND ORPHANAGE. This edifice dates back to 1868, and it was made possible by an endowment from Mrs. A.C. Caniff and others. It was a home for the sick, aged, and poor. It was run by St. Paul's Episcopalian Church, but people of all religions were admitted. (Courtesy Burton Historical Collection, Detroit Public Library.)

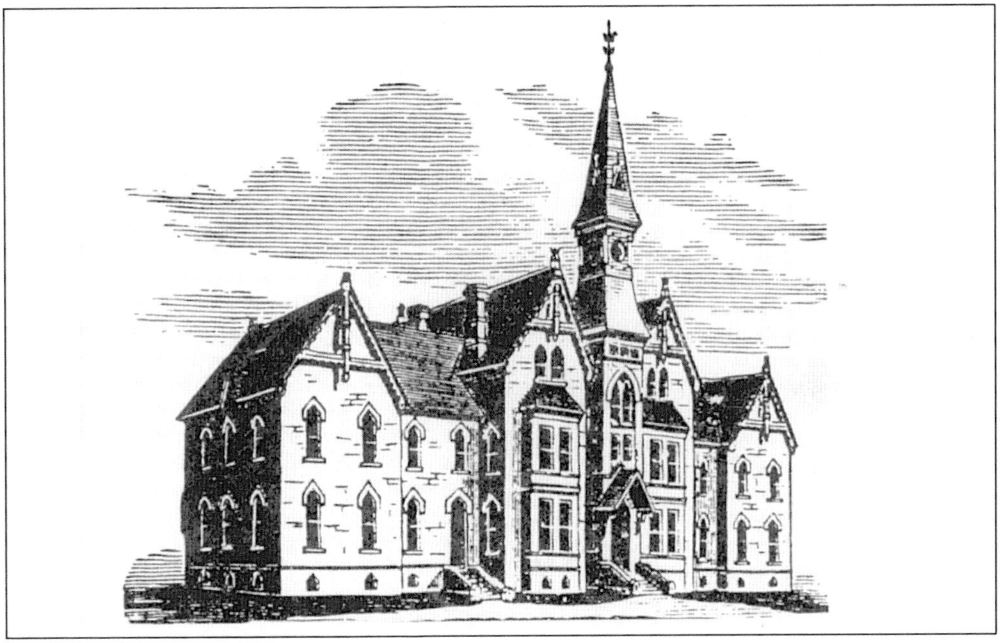

HOME OF THE FRIENDLESS, c. 1874. As the name implies, this was a home for friendless and homeless women and children. It also cared for children of mothers who were widows or worked as servants. The building was on the south side of Warren near Woodward Avenue. There are no known extant photos of this building. This drawing is from Farmer's *History of Detroit and Wayne County and Early Michigan*.

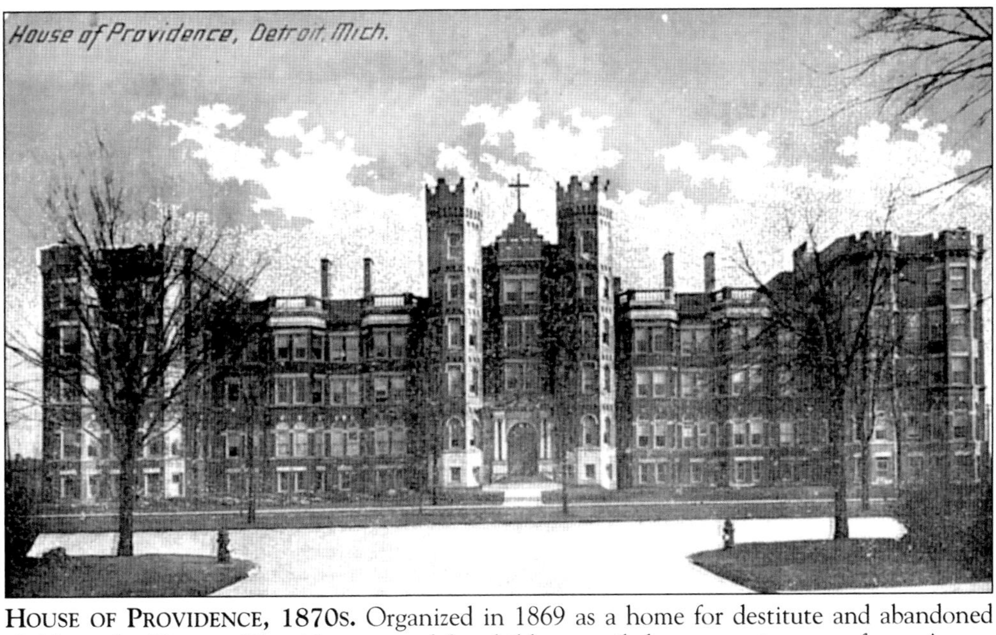

HOUSE OF PROVIDENCE, 1870S. Organized in 1869 as a home for destitute and abandoned children, the House of Providence cared for children until they were six years of age. At age six they were either given up for adoption or transferred to an orphan asylum. It was run by the Daughters of Charity, and the building was converted into Providence Hospital in 1910. There were apartments in the hospital for unwed mothers and their children.

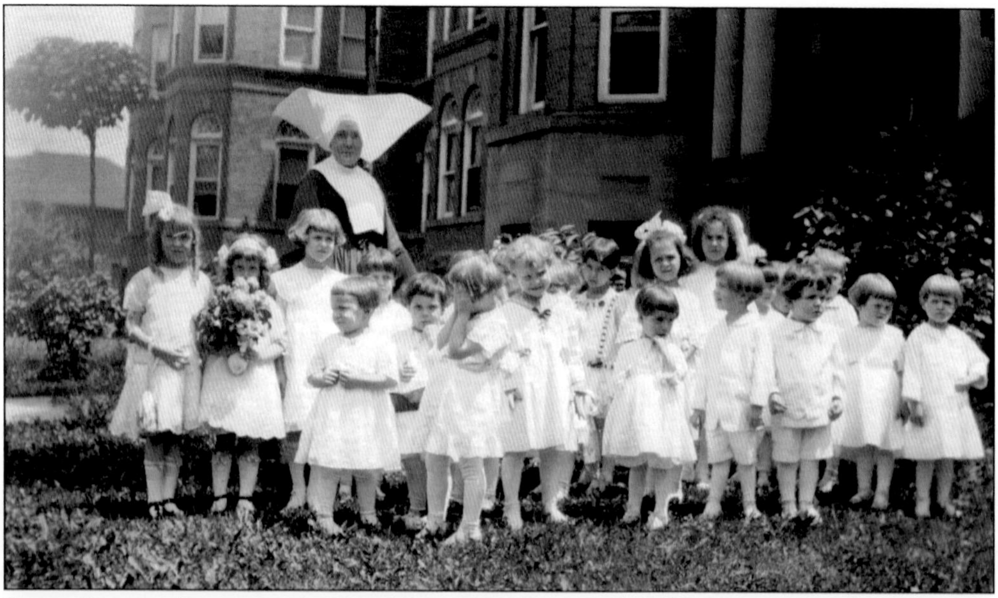

SISTER OLYMPIA BRADLEY AND CHILDREN, 1927. Sister is posed front of the House of Providence with some children who are dressed in their Sunday best for a special occasion, possibly the celebration of Easter. One of the children is camera shy and is covering her face with her hands. (Courtesy Daughters of Charity Archives, Mater Dei Provincialate, Evansville, Indiana.)

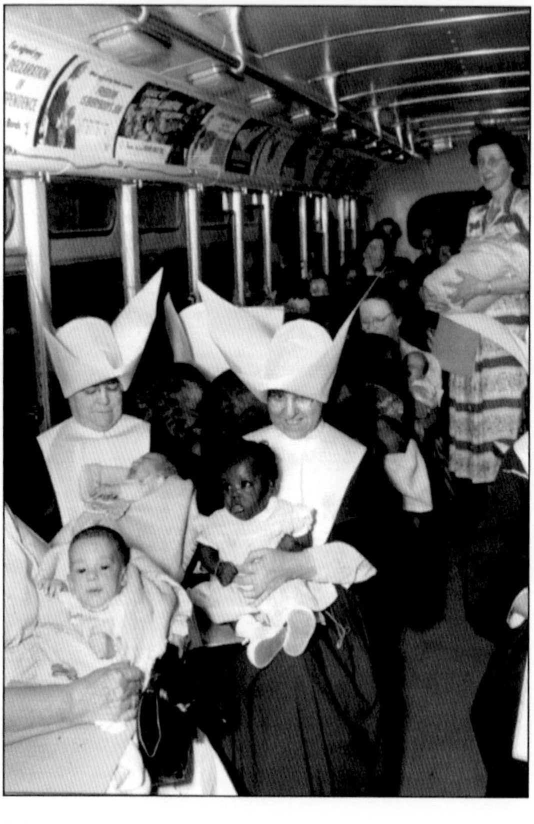

MOVING TO THE ST. VINCENT AND SARAH FISHER HOME, FARMINGTON HILLS, 1950. Two Daughters of Charity, Sr. Martina Murry (left) and Sr. Rita, and volunteers are shown taking children from Providence Hospital to the new St. Vincent and Sarah Fischer Home on August 10, 1950. This home cared for children from infancy through the teen years. (Courtesy Daughters of Charity Archives, Mater Dei Provincialate, Evansville, Indiana.)

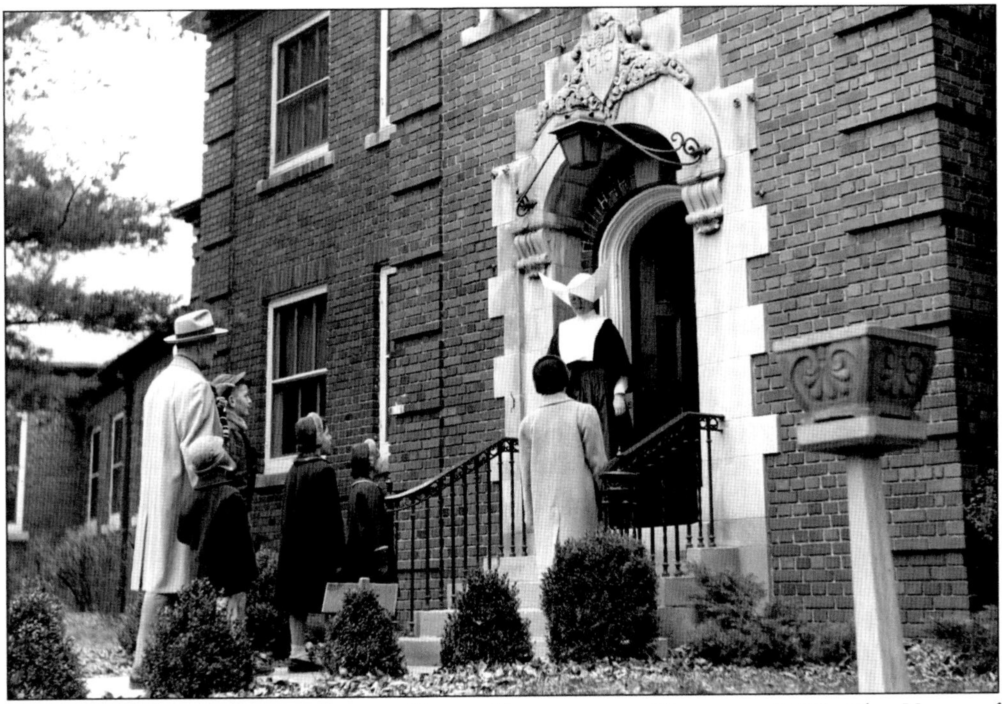

St. Vincent and Sarah Fisher Home, Farmington Hills, c. 1955. The House of Providence evolved into the St. Vincent and Sarah Fisher Home in Farmington Hills. Sister Blanche Culligan greets a family on the porch of the home which opened in 1929 on 80 acres on the northwest corner of 12 Mile and Inkster Roads. (Courtesy Daughters of Charity Archives, Mater Dei Provincialate, Evansville, Indiana.)

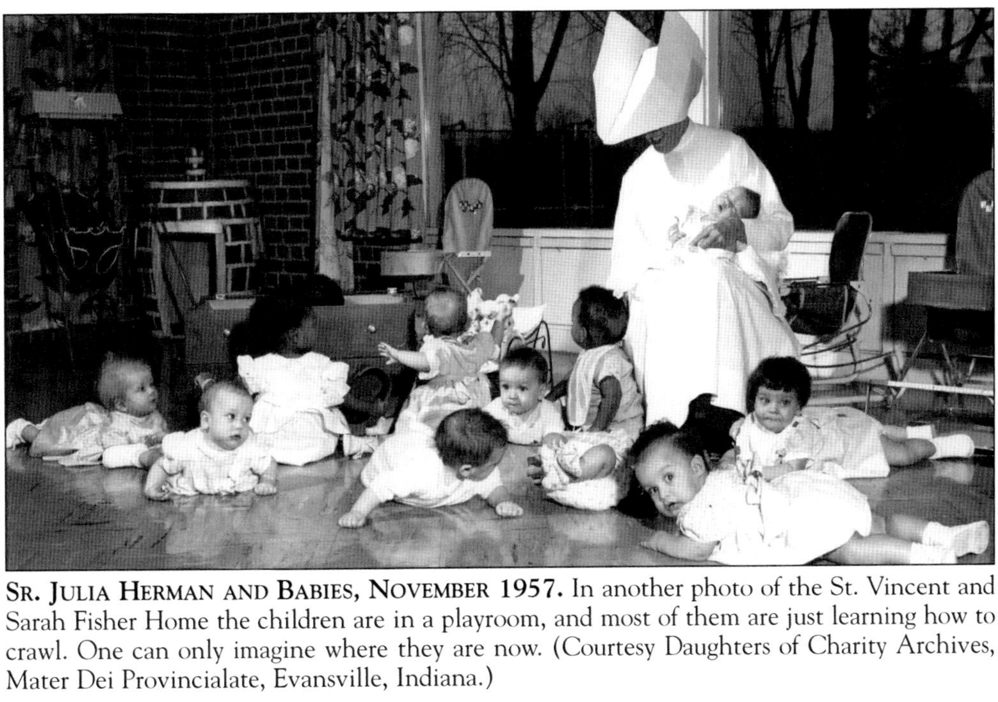

Sr. Julia Herman and Babies, November 1957. In another photo of the St. Vincent and Sarah Fisher Home the children are in a playroom, and most of them are just learning how to crawl. One can only imagine where they are now. (Courtesy Daughters of Charity Archives, Mater Dei Provincialate, Evansville, Indiana.)

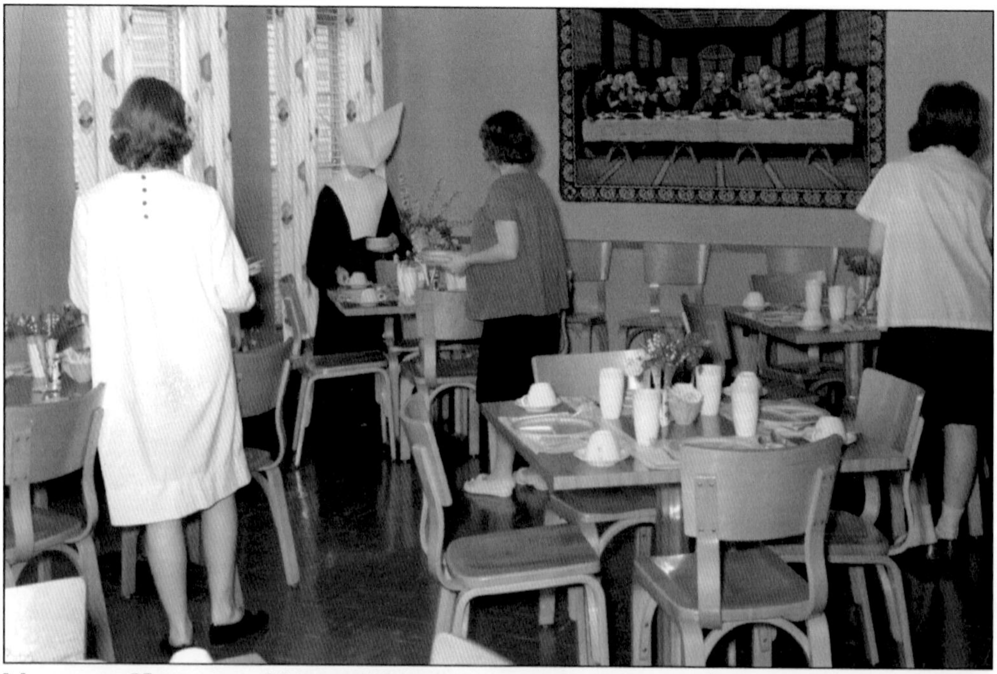

Marillac Hall for Unwed Mothers, Farmington, 1958. In 1953 the Marillac Apartments became the new home for unwed mothers. These young women are shown in the dining room of the facility. This residential program was discontinued in 1991. (Courtesy Daughters of Charity Archives, Mater Dei Provincialate, Evansville, Indiana.)

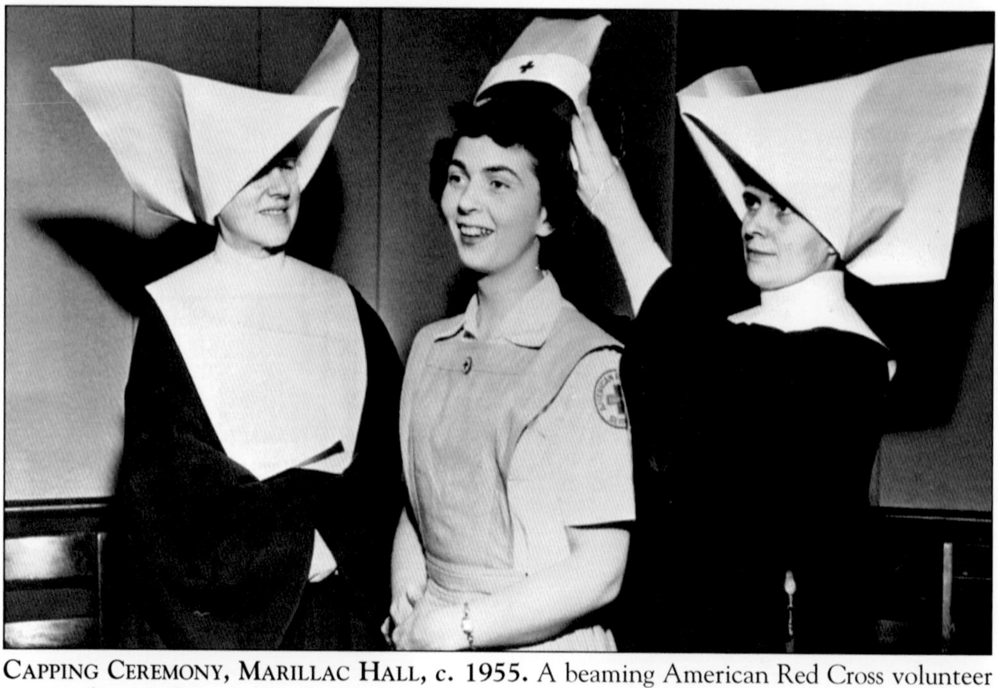

Capping Ceremony, Marillac Hall, c. 1955. A beaming American Red Cross volunteer is given her cap by two Daughters of Charity after successfully completing a training program. (Courtesy Daughters of Charity Archives, Mater Dei Provincialate, Evansville, Indiana.)

THE THOMPSON HOME FOR OLD LADIES, 2003. This stately Victorian home has survived for 110 years, probably because it was fortunate enough to be built on what is now the Wayne State University campus. This home evolved from the Home of the Friendless which was located nearby on Warren Avenue. Mrs. David (Mary) Thompson built the original structure in 1884 on Cass at Hancock. It was a home for genteel, aged women.

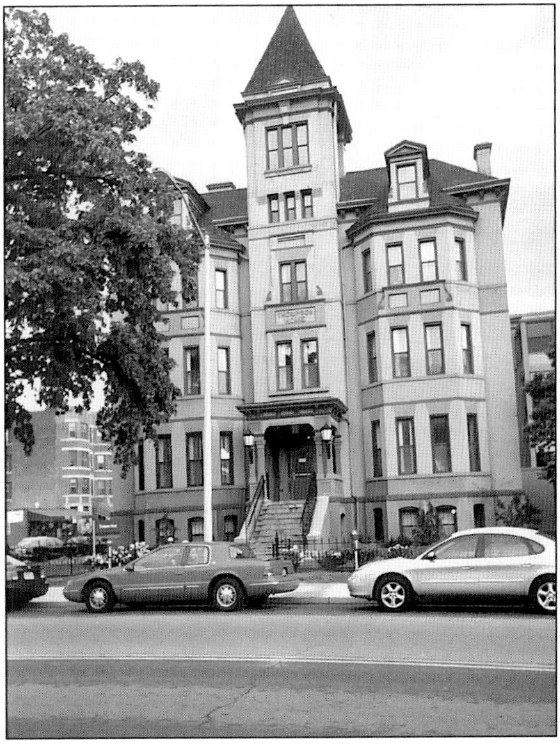

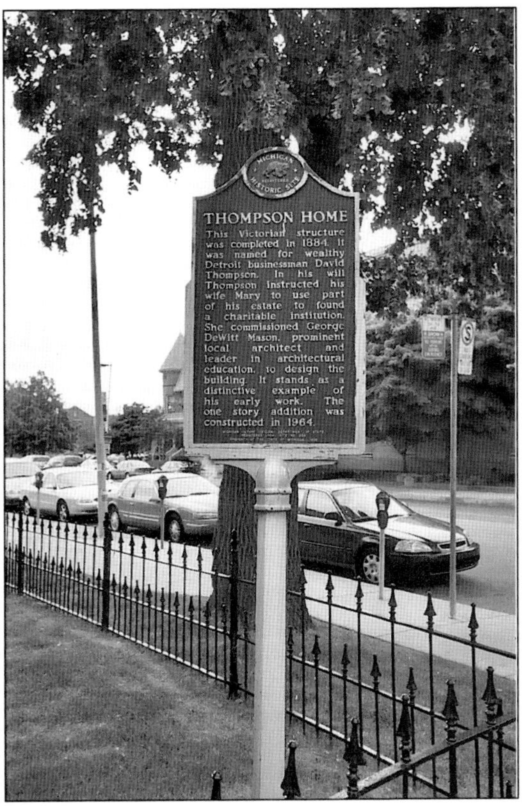
MICHIGAN
HISTORIC SITE
THOMPSON HOME
This Victorian structure was completed in 1884. It was named for wealthy Detroit businessman David Thompson. In his will Thompson instructed his wife Mary to use part of his estate to found a charitable institution. She commissioned George DeWitt Mason, prominent local architect and leader in architectural education, to design the building. It stands as a distinctive example of his early work. The one story addition was constructed in 1964.

HISTORIC MARKER, THOMPSON HOME. George DeWitt Mason, a prominent Detroit architect, designed this home. Mason also designed the First Presbyterian Church in Detroit, and the Grand Hotel on Mackinac Island. The building currently and appropriately houses Wayne State University's School of Social Work.

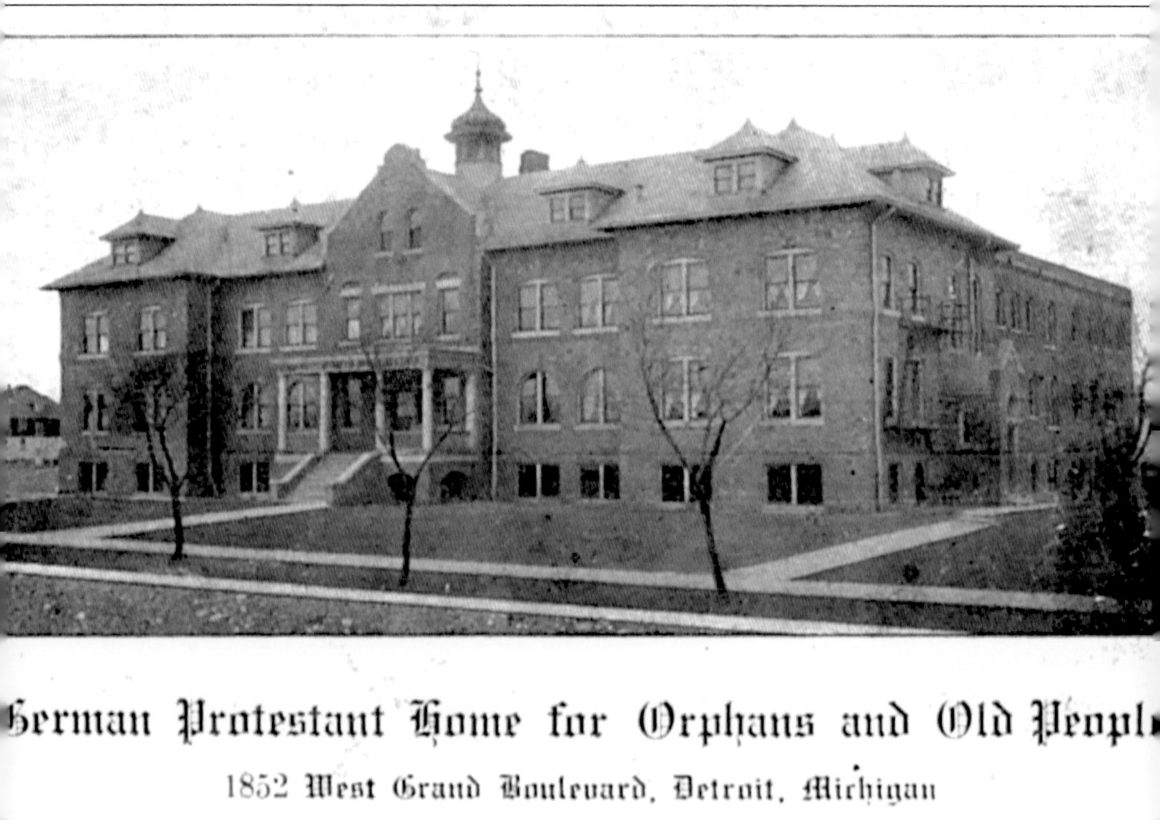

GERMAN PROTESTANT HOME FOR ORPHANS AND OLD PEOPLE, c. 1920. This home was located at 1852 West Grand Boulevard and was run by German Americans. The military fiction writer Hugo Matson and his sister were housed here during World War II. They weren't orphans, but their mother had to work, so she had no choice but to place them somewhere for care. She only made $20 a week, and spent $8 of that on room and board for her children. Matson remembers a strict atmosphere and lumpy oatmeal. Everyone went to chapel for two hours every morning, one hour of which was conducted in German. (Courtesy Cheryl Strange-Laetsch.)

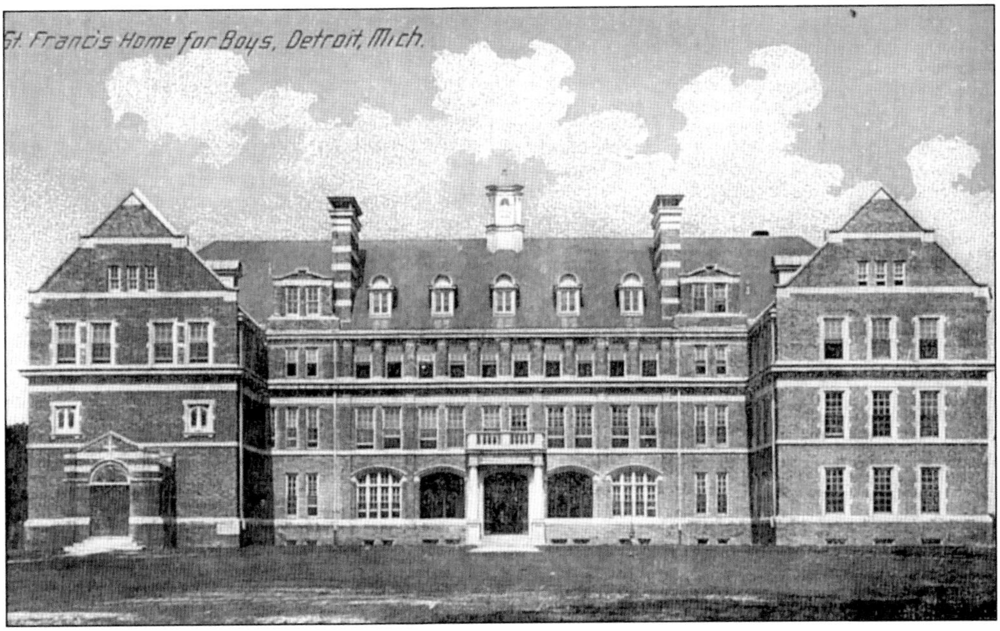

ST. FRANCIS HOME FOR BOYS. This orphanage was established in 1909 and is shown both in a postcard of that era and also as it appeared in the 1950s. The original building was on Woodward Avenue between Victor and Ferris in Highland Park. The facility is now located at 17500 West 8 Mile Road in Southfield. (Courtesy Archdiocese of Detroit.)

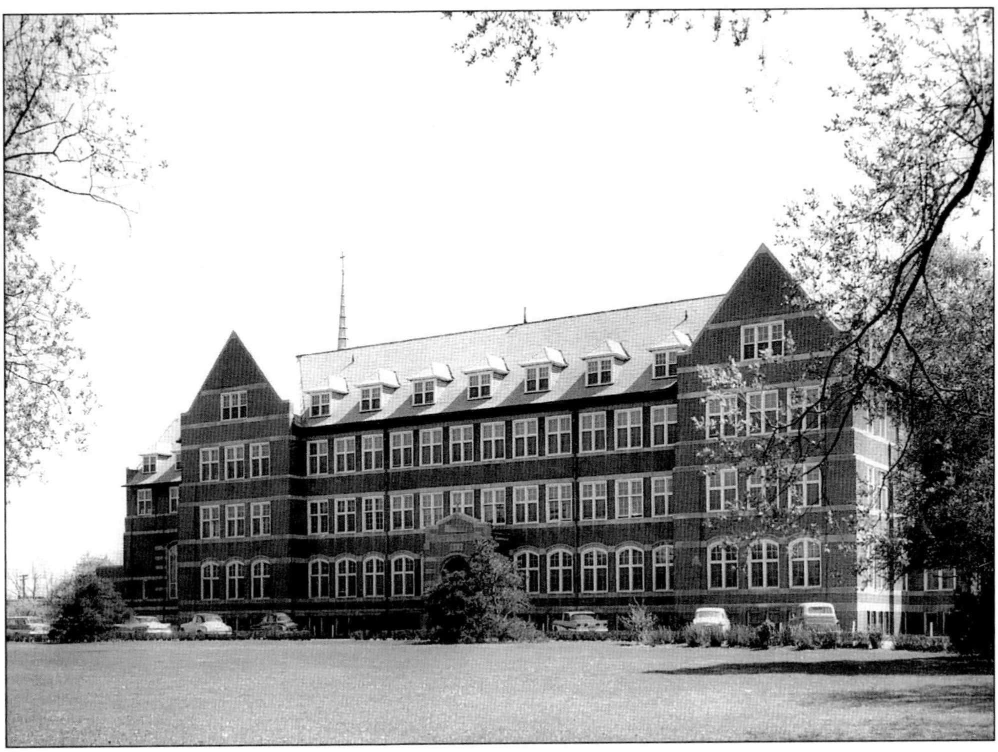

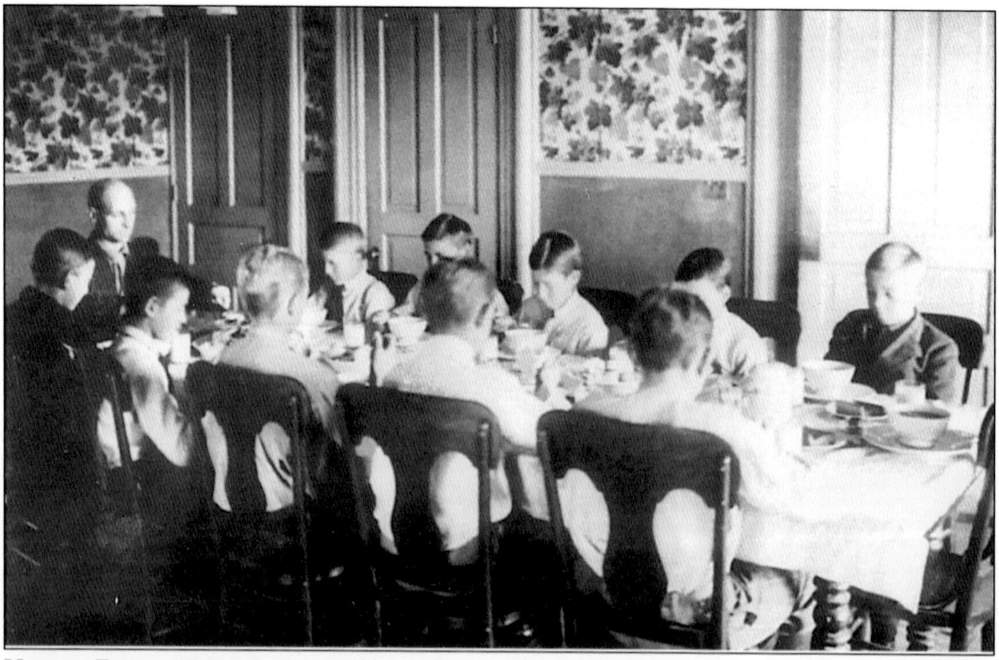

Valley Farm, 1911. A group of boys dine in this home built in 1861 by Alfred Gulley Sr. on the north side of Michigan Avenue near the present Gulley Road in Dearborn. Henry Ford bought the home and used it as a home for orphan boys. This facility was closed in 1916, and reopened in 1918 as an annex to Woman's Hospital. (Courtesy Dearborn Historical Museum.)

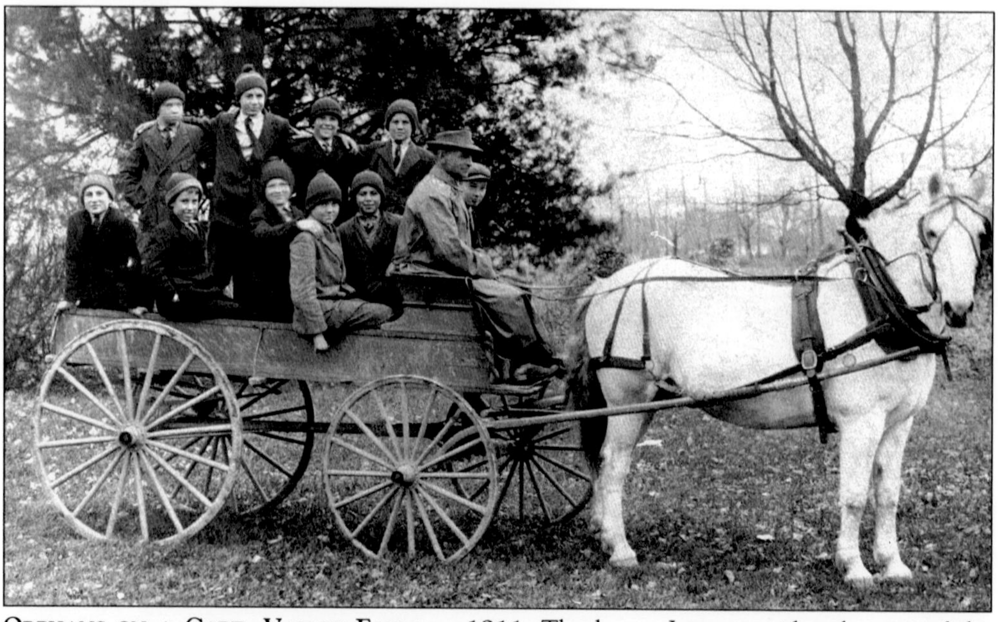

Orphans on a Cart, Valley Farm, c. 1911. The horse, Jerry, is said to be part of the original team owned by Henry Ford. The boys are identified, from left to right: (top) Stanley Woski, Morris Smit, Jerome Heytens, John Gries, Daniel Lorimer (seated by driver), and August Barth, the driver and manager; (bottom) George Brady, Jesse Bollinger, Lewis Brady, Walter Fink, and Herbert Smit. (Courtesy Dearborn Historical Museum.)

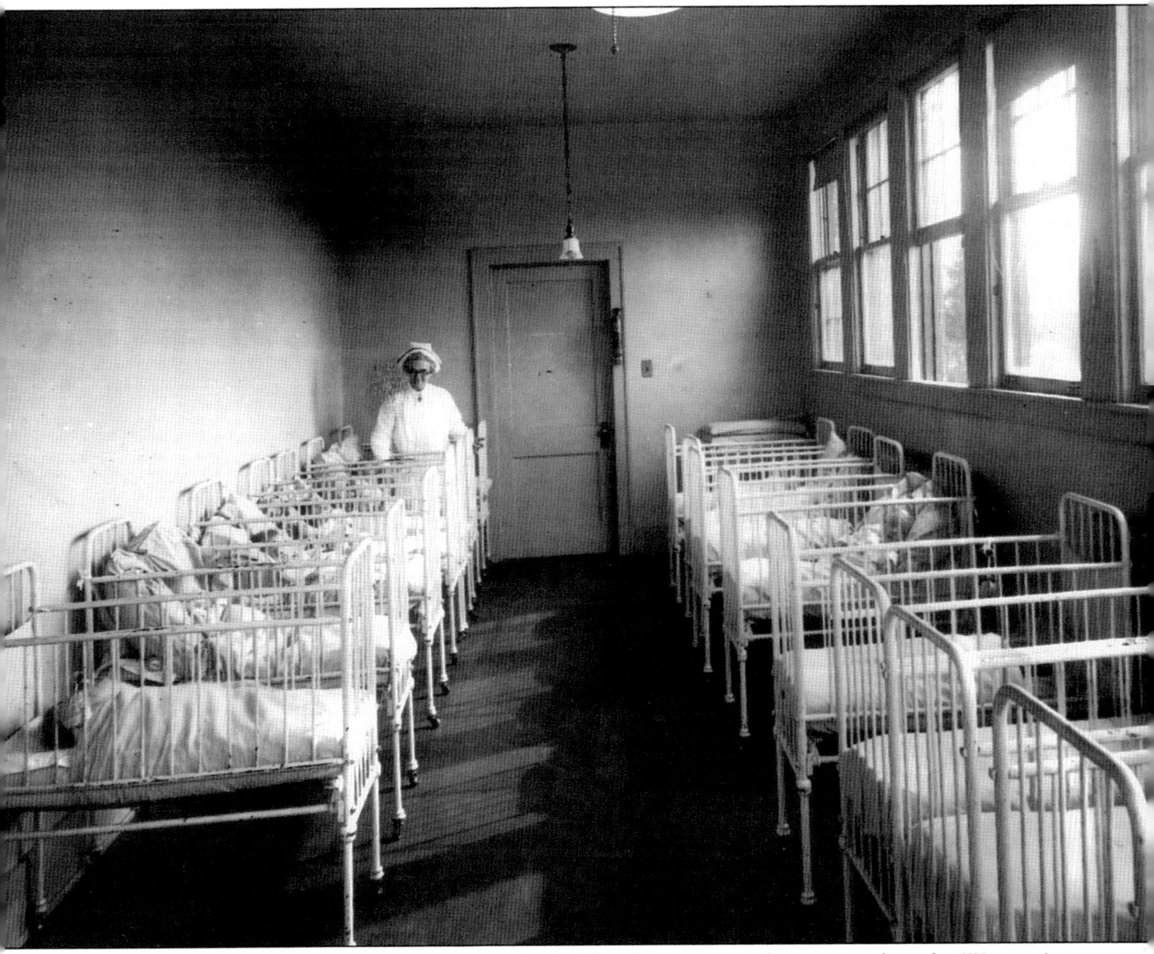

NURSERY, VALLEY FARM, DEARBORN, c. 1918. This farm was used as an auxiliary by Woman's Hospital to take care of young women euphemistically referred to as "fallen by the way" before and after the birth of their babies. A nurse stands watch over her little patients in this rather austere and rustic nursery. Their mothers tended gardens, canned produce, and made embroidered pieces to sell which produced an income for them of $3 to $5 per week. Most of the women went into domestic service, and they took their babies with them when they left Valley Farm. (Courtesy Dearborn Historical Museum.)

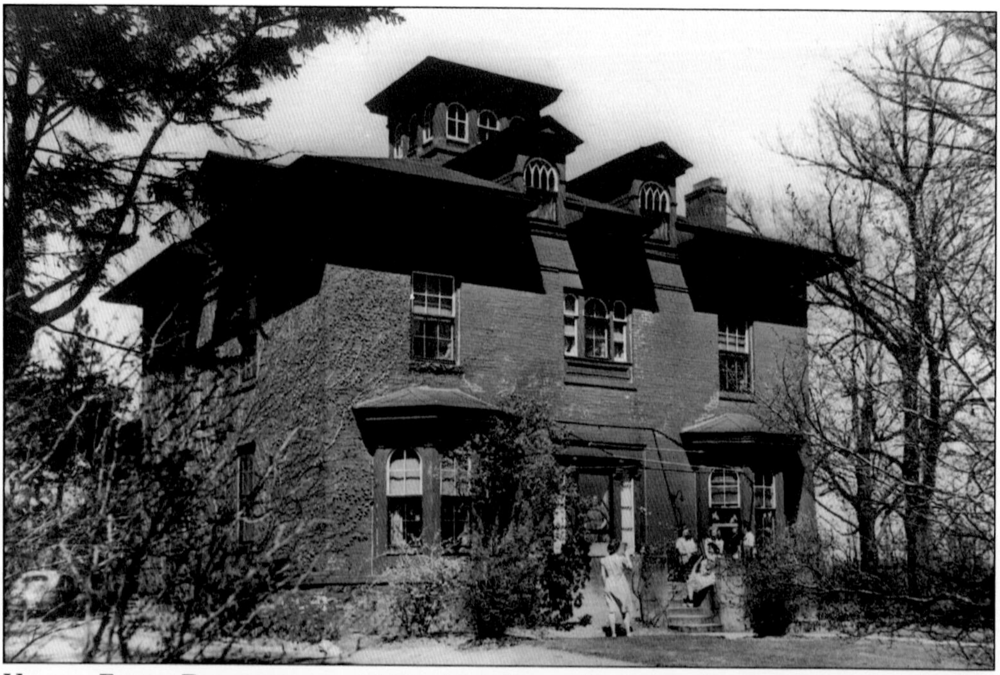

VALLEY FARM, DEARBORN, c. 1940s. Mrs. Henry Ford donated the house and land to Woman's Hospital, and also paid for repairs. The Benevolent Protective Order of Elks acquired the farm and home in 1955, and they removed the cupola and the second floor of the structure in 1970. This building is still there, but there is no resemblance to the original. (Courtesy Dearborn Historical Museum)

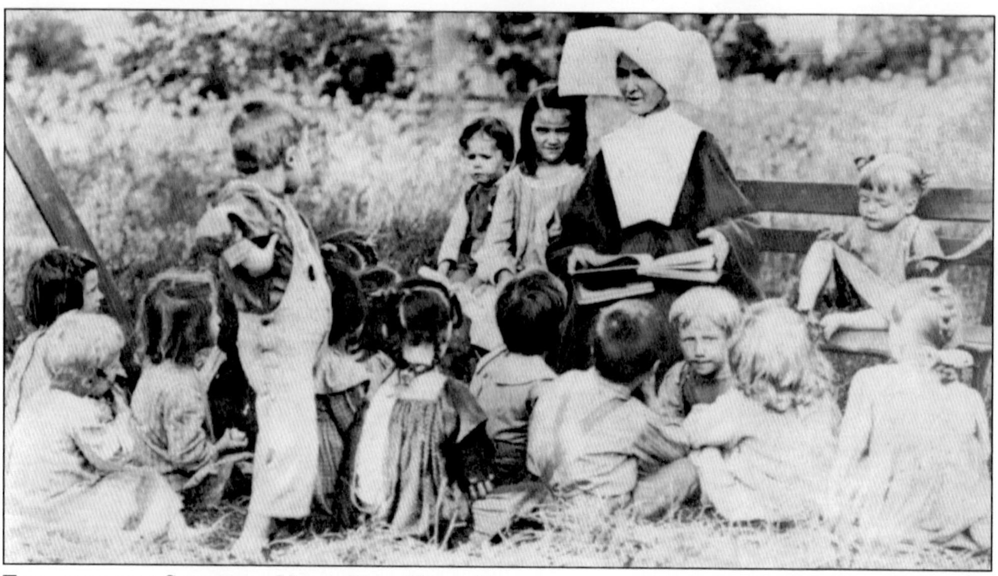

ENJOYING THE SHADE AT VILLA PAR-WELL, DEARBORN, c. 1920. In 1903, William Partridge and Henry Blackwell donated six acres of land in Dearborn Township with barns, a house, and orchards to be used by the orphans living at the House of Providence. Here a Daughter of Charity reads to a group of children. (Courtesy Daughter of Charity Archives, Mater Dei Provincialate, Evansville, Indiana.)

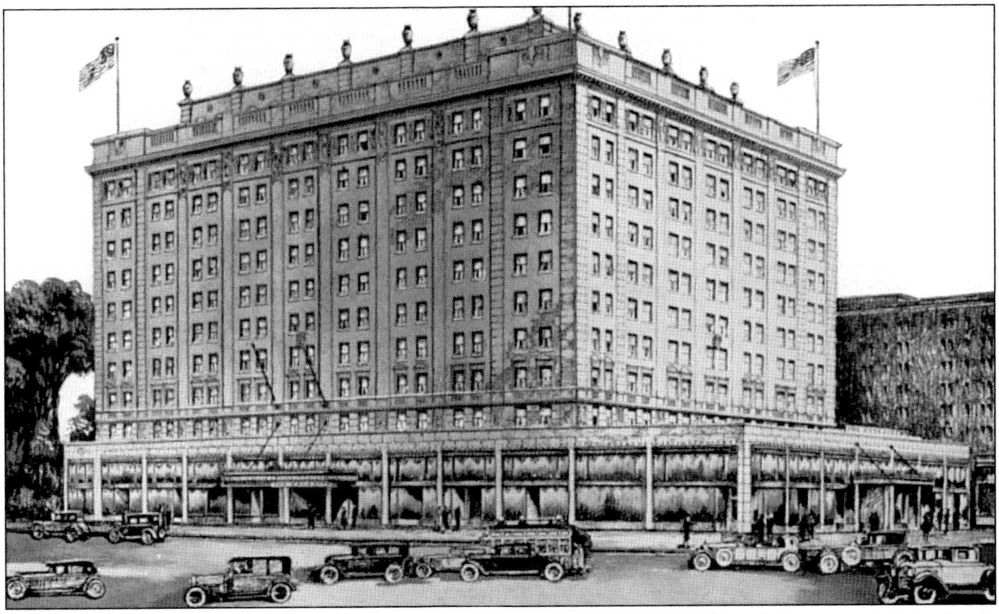

THE DETROITER, 1930S. This is a postcard of the hotel built as the Hotel Savoy in 1926, which later became the Hotel LaSalle. It was renamed the Detroiter by 1931. It was 12 stories high and had 800 rooms, 18 corner suites, and a two-story penthouse apartment. It was designed by the well-known architect Louis Kemper and was located at Woodward Avenue and Adelaide.

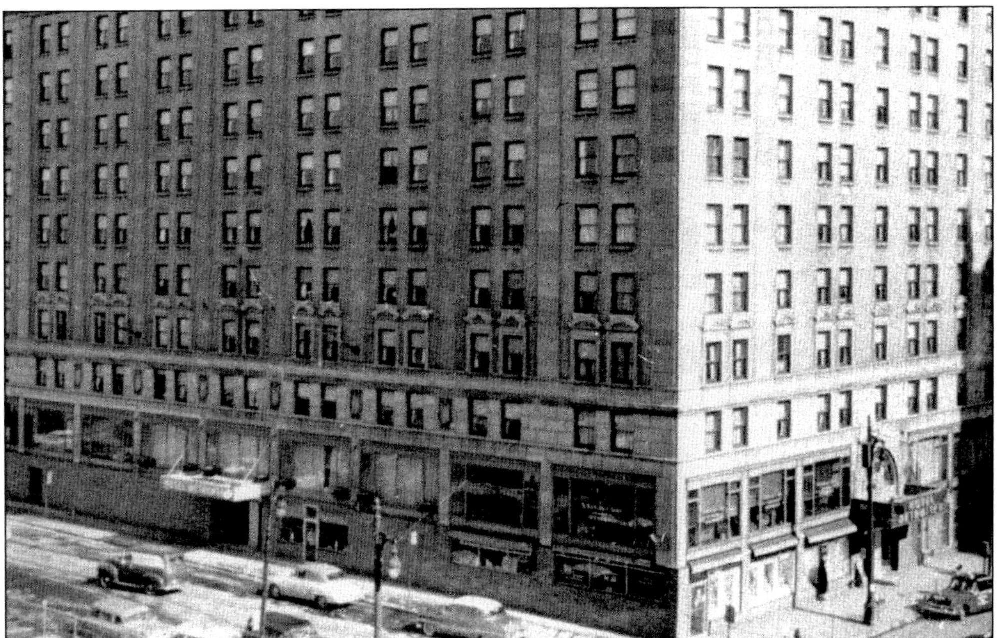

THE DETROITER/CARMEL HALL, 1950S. This is how the hotel looked just before it became Carmel Hall in 1955. Carmel Hall was a residence for the elderly that was operated by the Carmelite Sisters of the Sick and Infirm, of Germantown, New York. Medical care was provided for residents, and meals were served in a community dining room. This type of facility was then a new concept for retired Detroiters. (Courtesy Archdiocese of Detroit.)

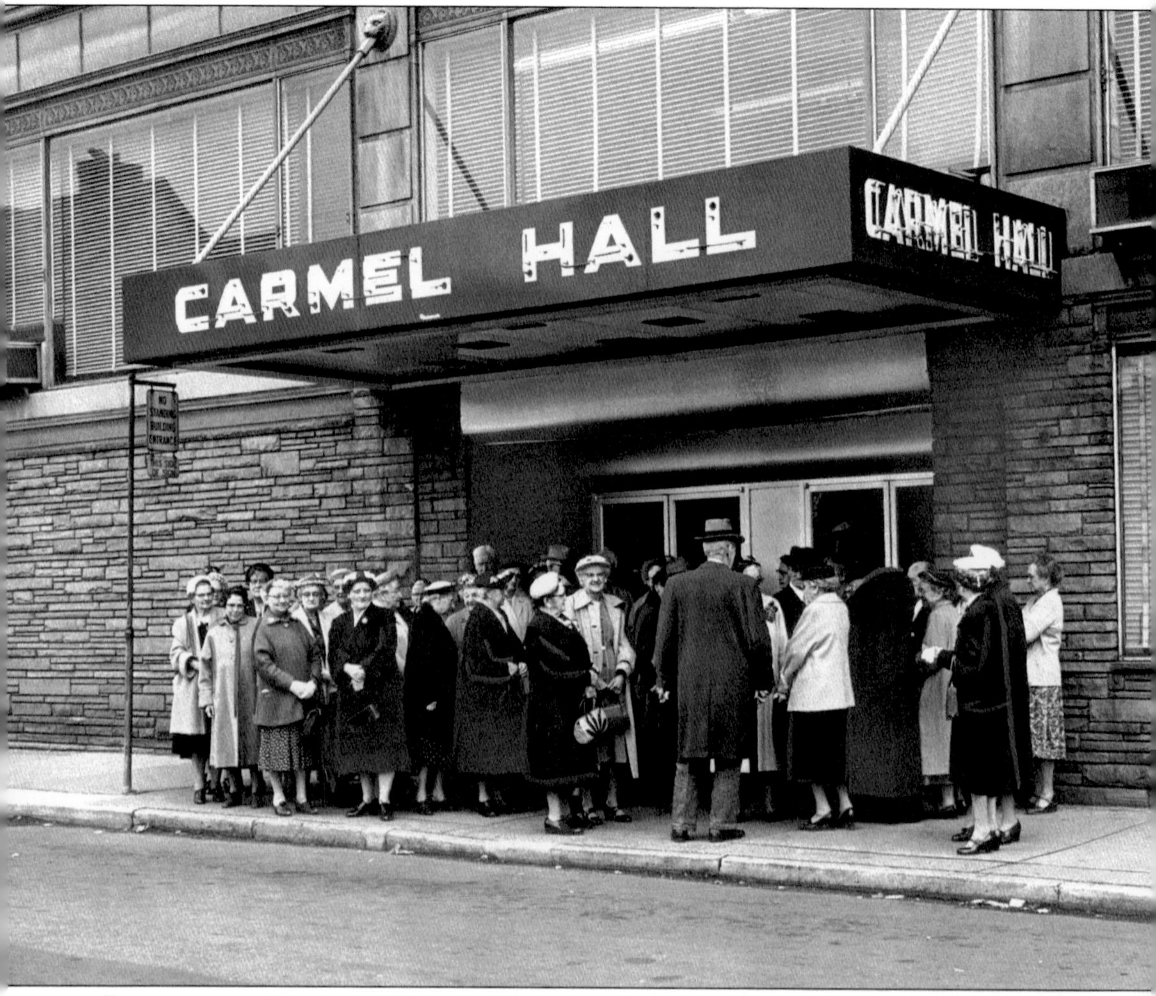

Residents in Front of Carmel Hall, c. 1960. A group of residents of Carmel Hall are awaiting transportation to the Holy Redeemer school auditorium to see a student performance of the play "The Gondoliers." The school put on a special matinee performance, and arranged transportation for the residents with a police-escorted motorcade. This building was imploded March 2, 1996, and new townhouses have been constructed on this site. (Courtesy Archdiocese of Detroit.)

Six

Now Just a Memory

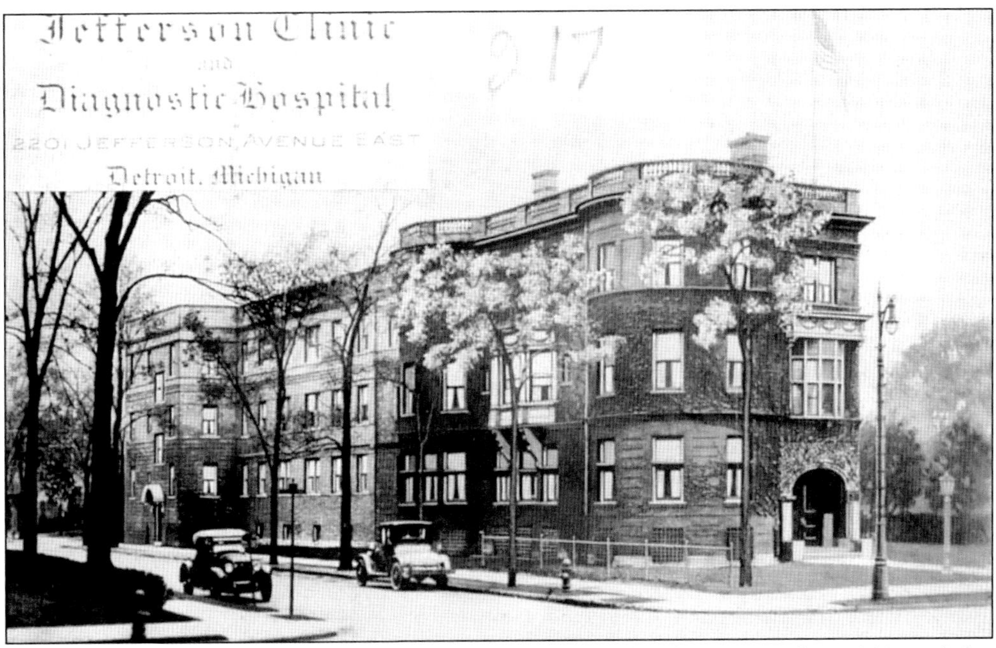

Jefferson Clinic and Diagnostic Hospital, 1925. The clinic opened in 1911, and this 50-bed general hospital opened in 1924 and was located at 2001 Jefferson Avenue East. In 1927, Carl I. Johnson was the superintendent and there were two resident physicians and one intern on staff. (Courtesy Cheryl Strange-Laetsch.)

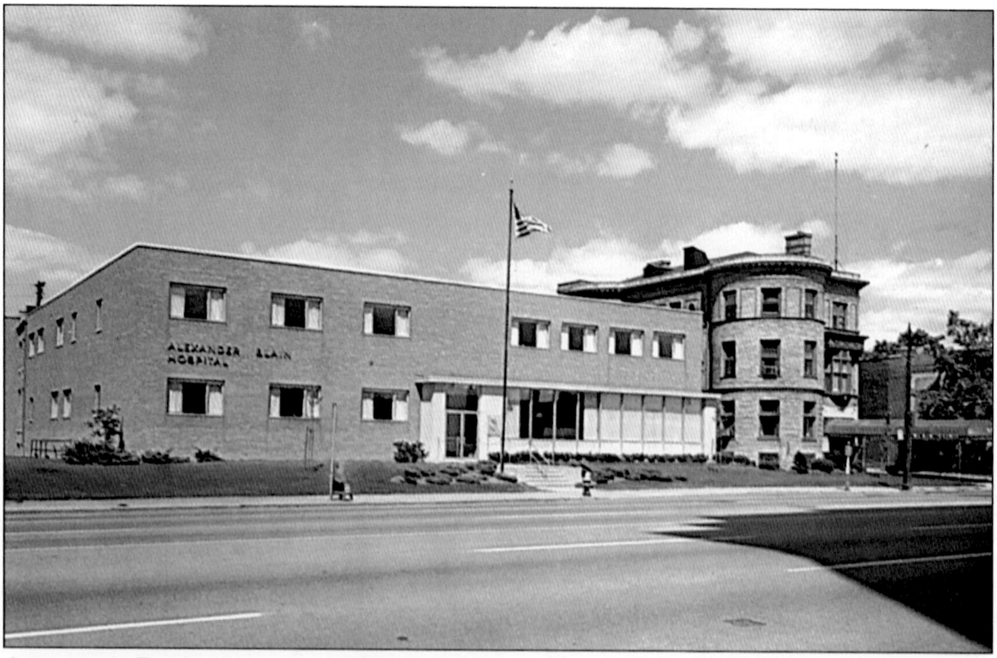

ALEXANDER BLAIN HOSPITAL, 1950S. Here is the Jefferson Clinic and Diagnostic Hospital after it was remodeled and renamed the Alexander Blain Hospital. Alexander W. Blain (1885–1958) was a surgeon and a conservationist. He helped establish the Michigan Audubon Society. The hospital is now part of the St. John Health System. (Courtesy Cheryl Strange-Laetsch.)

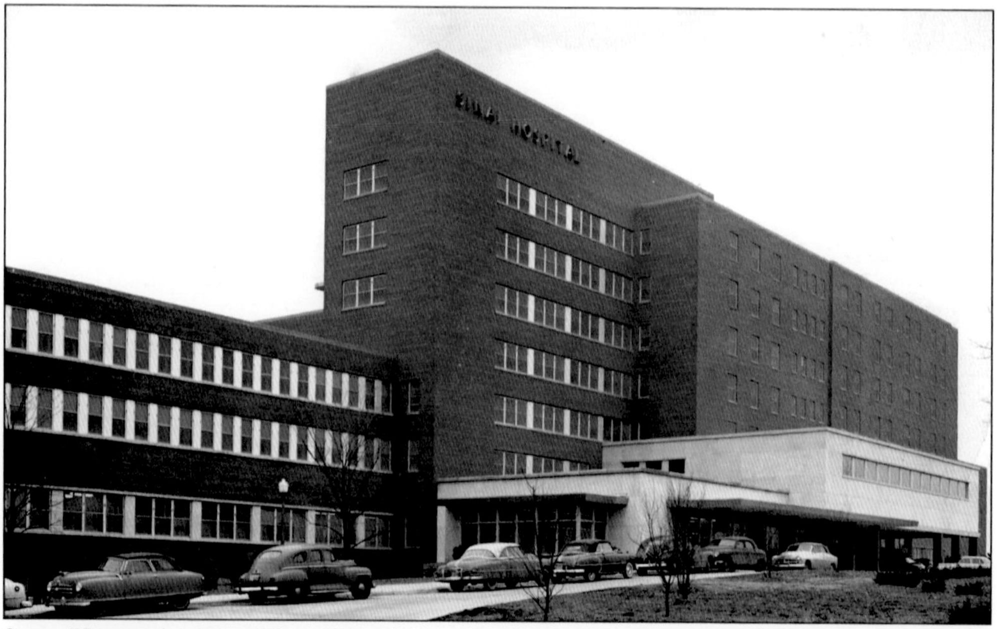

SINAI HOSPITAL, 1950. This is how the 211-bed, pavilion-type hospital looked when it opened in January 1953. It was the second hospital to be completed under the Greater Detroit Hospital fund, and it primarily served the Jewish community in metropolitan Detroit. It offered patients the services of a rabbi, Kosher meals, and the observance of Jewish holidays and traditions. (Courtesy Burton Historical Collection, Detroit Public Library.)

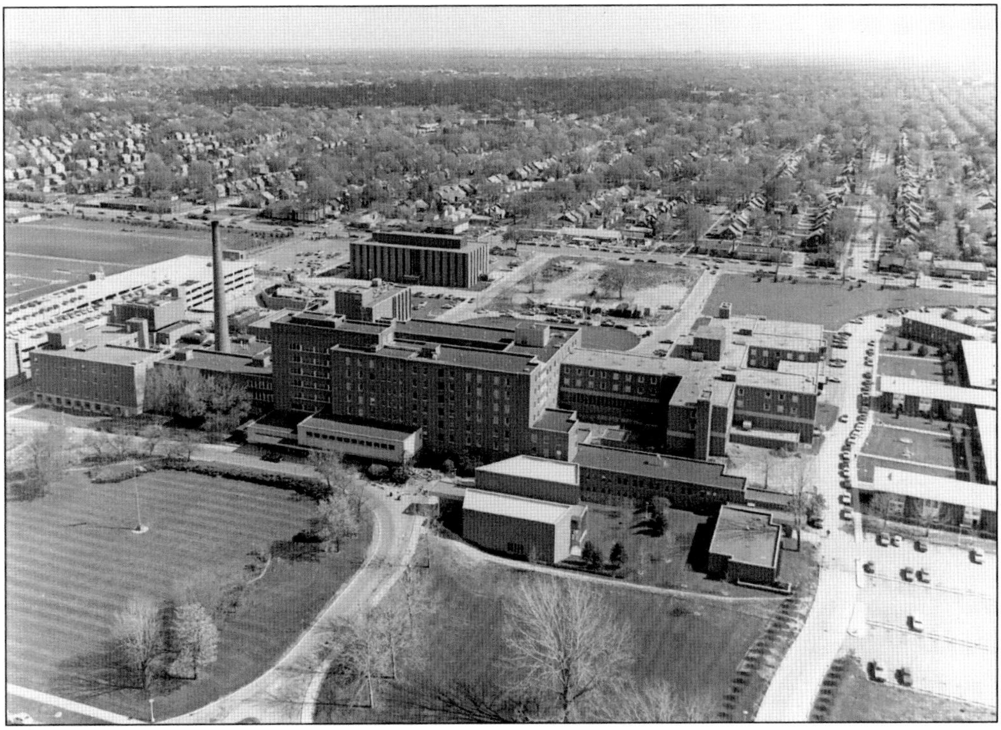

SINAI HOSPITAL, AERIAL VIEW. The hospital grew considerably in size and eventually became a large complex at 6767 W. Outer Drive. The hospital merged with Grace to form Sinai Grace Hospital in the Detroit Medical Center. The center closed in September of 1999 and sits vacant. (Courtesy Leonard N. Simons Jewish Community Archives, Walter P. Reuther Library, Wayne State University.)

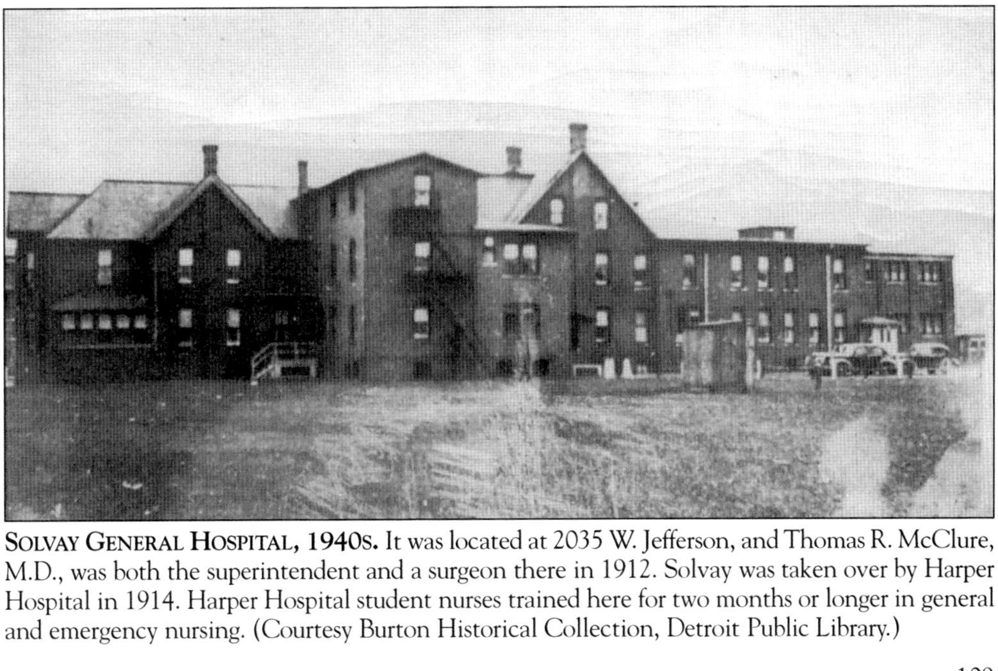

SOLVAY GENERAL HOSPITAL, 1940S. It was located at 2035 W. Jefferson, and Thomas R. McClure, M.D., was both the superintendent and a surgeon there in 1912. Solvay was taken over by Harper Hospital in 1914. Harper Hospital student nurses trained here for two months or longer in general and emergency nursing. (Courtesy Burton Historical Collection, Detroit Public Library.)

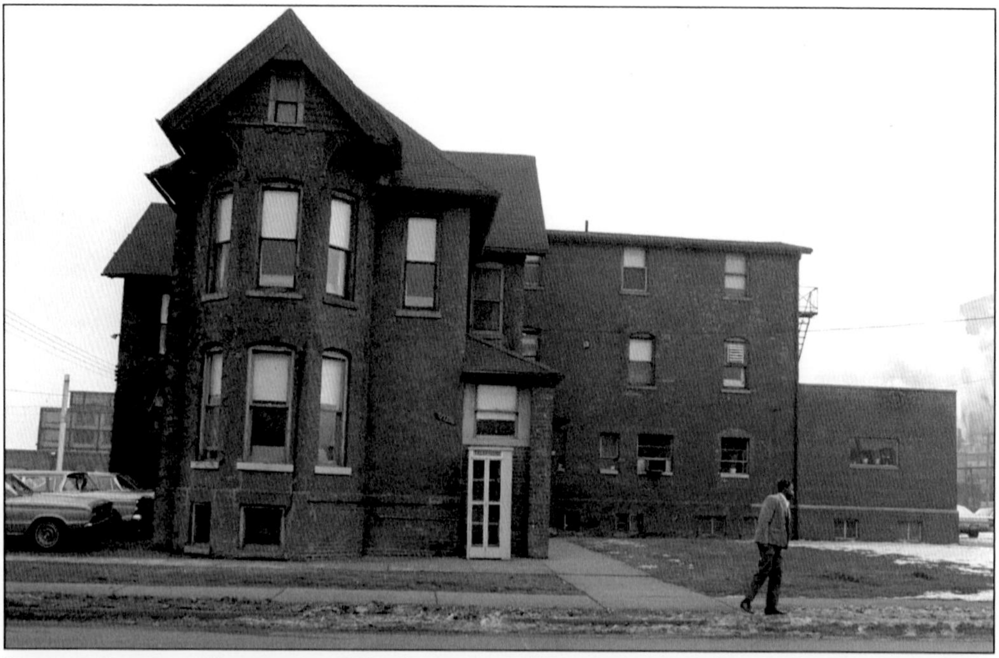

DELRAY GENERAL HOSPITAL, 1967. A man is walking in front of the 105-bed hospital which was located at 7125 West Jefferson in the Delray area of Detroit. It was originally the industrial clinic for the Solvay Process Company. It was later part of a four-way hospital merger to become the new Southwest General Hospital, which closed in 1991. (Courtesy Walter P. Reuther Library, Wayne State University.)

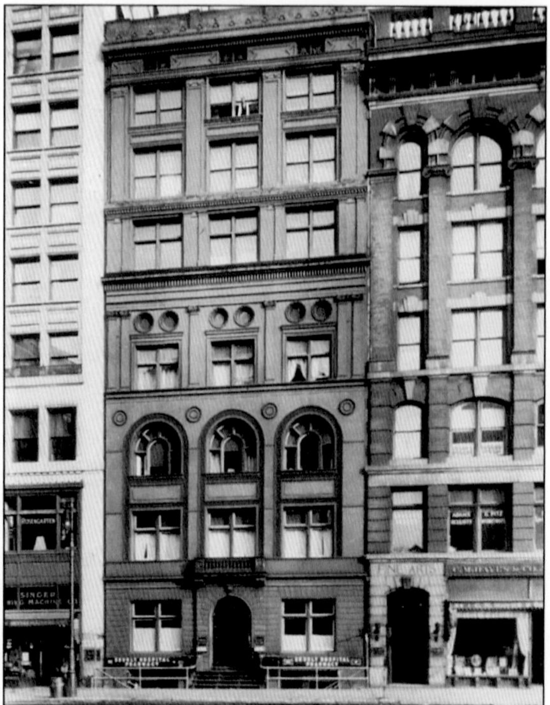

DETROIT EYE, EAR, NOSE, AND THROAT HOSPITAL, 1927. It was also called Shurly Hospital after its Chief of Staff, Burt R. Shurly, M.D. The building was located in downtown Detroit at 62 W. Adams, and had a bed capacity of 120 patients. The hospital rate included only liquid food. There was a hospital pharmacy which was open to the public. (Courtesy Burton Historical Collection, Detroit Public Library)

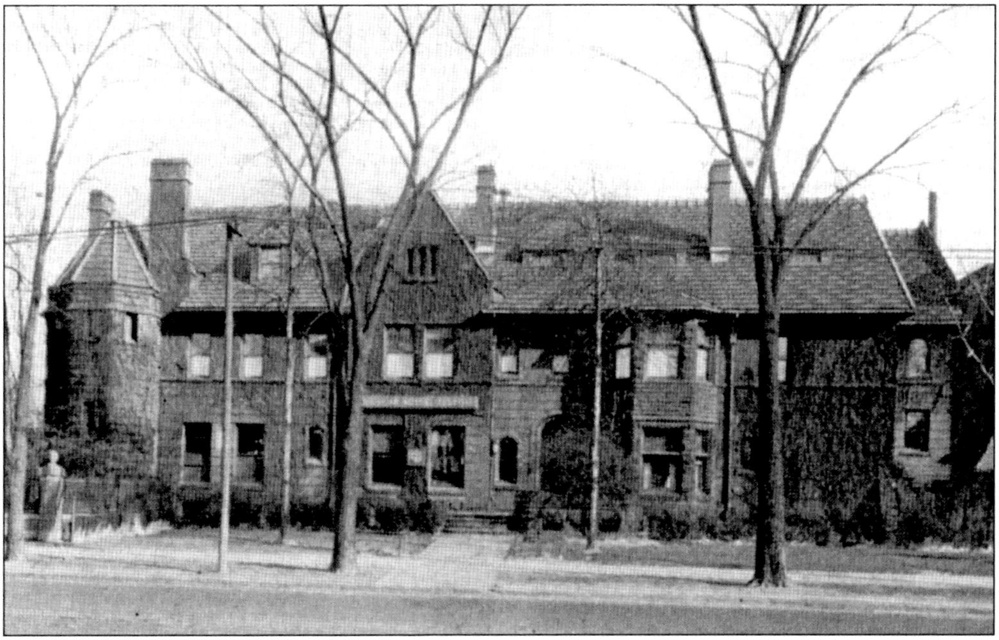

Michigan Mutual Hospital, c. 1927. Located at 2730 E. Jefferson, this was an industrial hospital with a bed capacity of 35. It was operated by the Michigan Mutual Liability Company. It treated injuries, and offered physical and occupational therapy

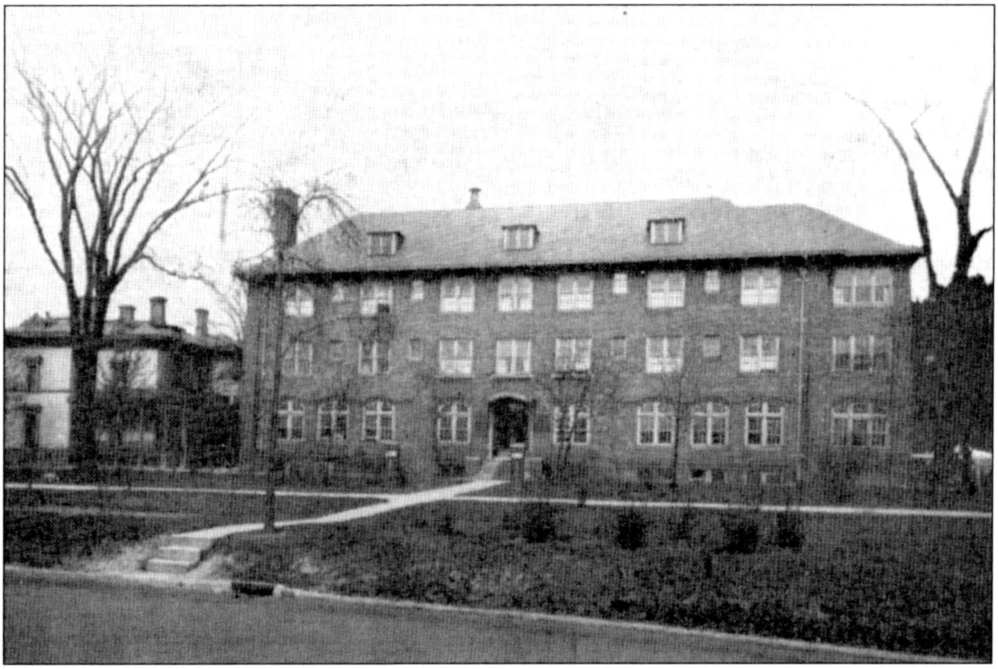

William Booth Memorial Home and Hospital, c. 1927. The Salvation Army ran this 20-bed maternity hospital for unwed mothers at 130 W. Grand Boulevard.

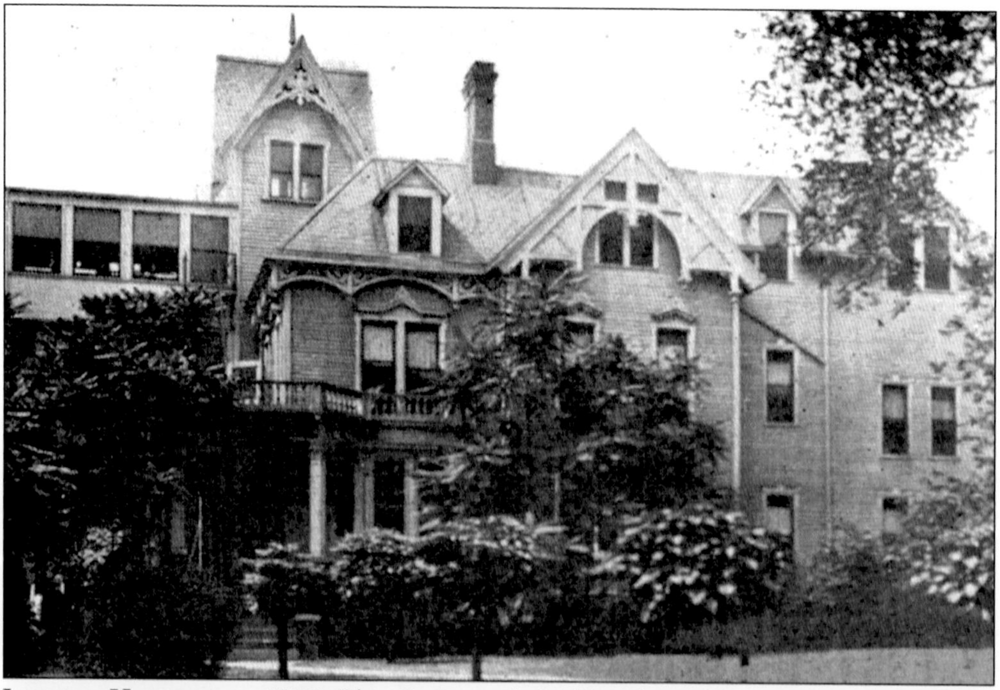

LINCOLN HOSPITAL, c. 1927. This Gothic style building housed a 50-bed general hospital which was located at 1051 Twenty-fifth Street.

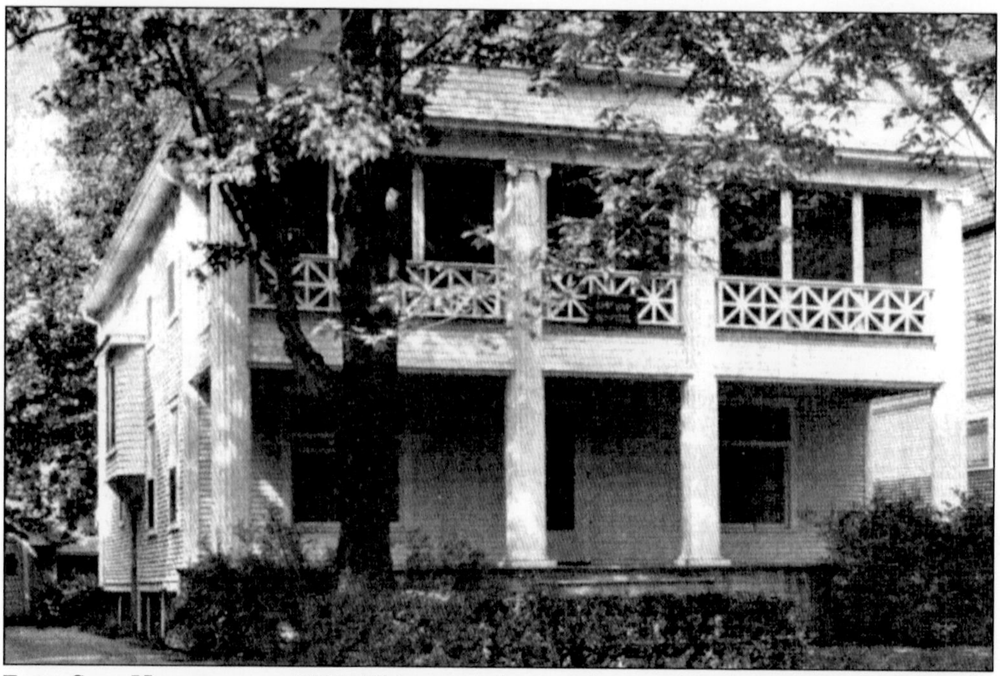

EAST SIDE HOSPITAL, c. 1927. This privately-owned surgical and maternity hospital was located at 2191–2199 Cadillac Boulevard. It had a bed capacity of 35. In 1927, the officer in charge and the governing body was one person—Minnie May Anderson, R.N. This hospital looked like a Southern plantation house, and it had a homey atmosphere.

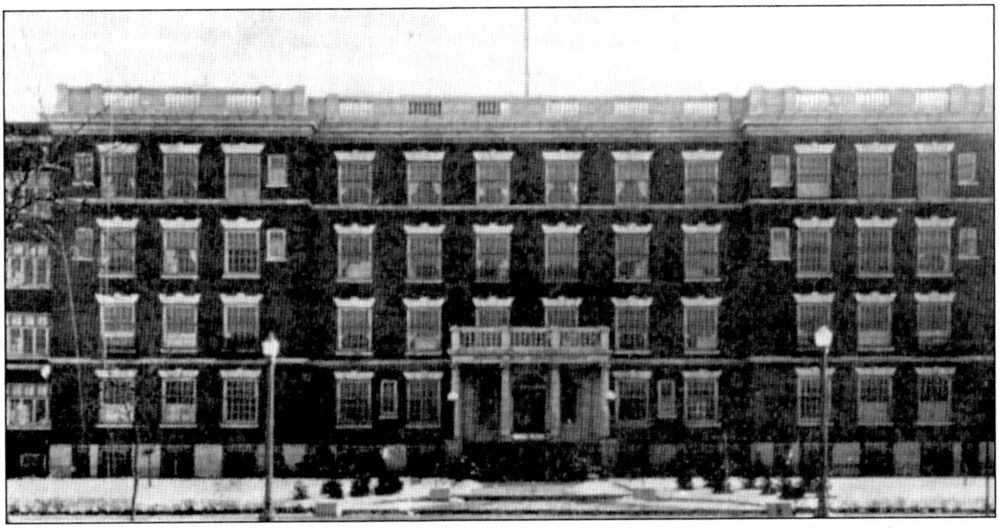

HIGHLAND PARK GENERAL HOSPITAL, c. 1927. Located at Glendale and Lincoln Avenue in Highland Park, this hospital had 150 beds and also ran a school of nursing. It opened in 1918, but did not open for patients until 1921. It treated psychiatric and contagious cases in addition to being a general hospital. It closed in 1976. The building was placed on the National Register of Historic Places in 1985. It was rehabilitated into a senior citizen complex called the Highland Park Apartments in 1988.

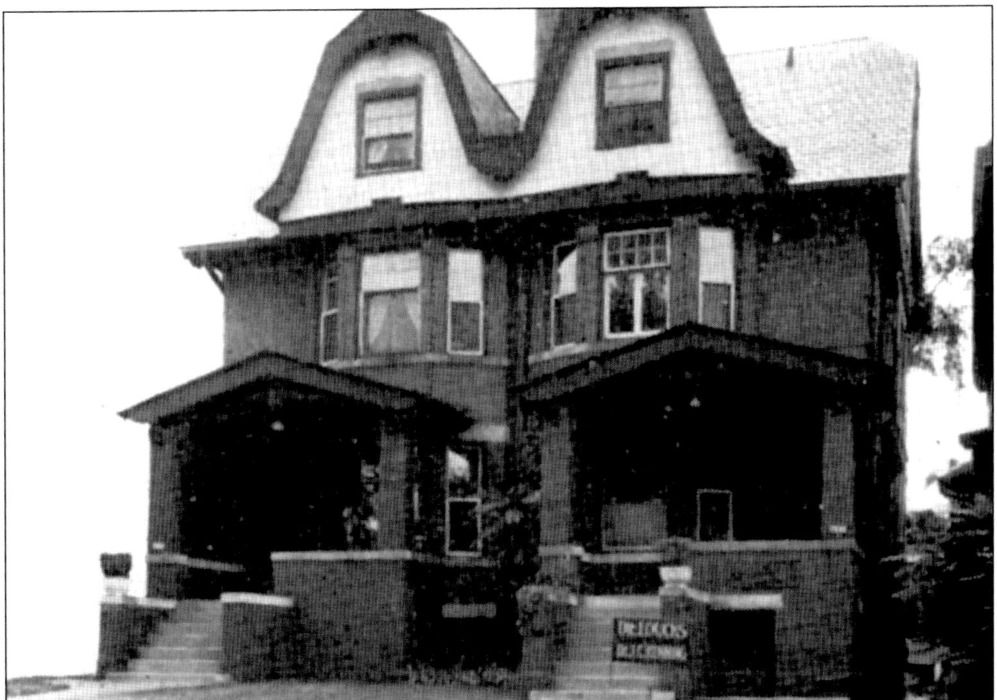

MEMORIAL HOSPITAL, c. 1927. Memorial was a popular name for hospitals, and Detroit had several. This one only had seven beds, and it was located at 337 West Grand Boulevard. It was used for radiation therapy for patients with cancer and thyroid problems. The doctor in charge was R.E. Loucks, M.D.

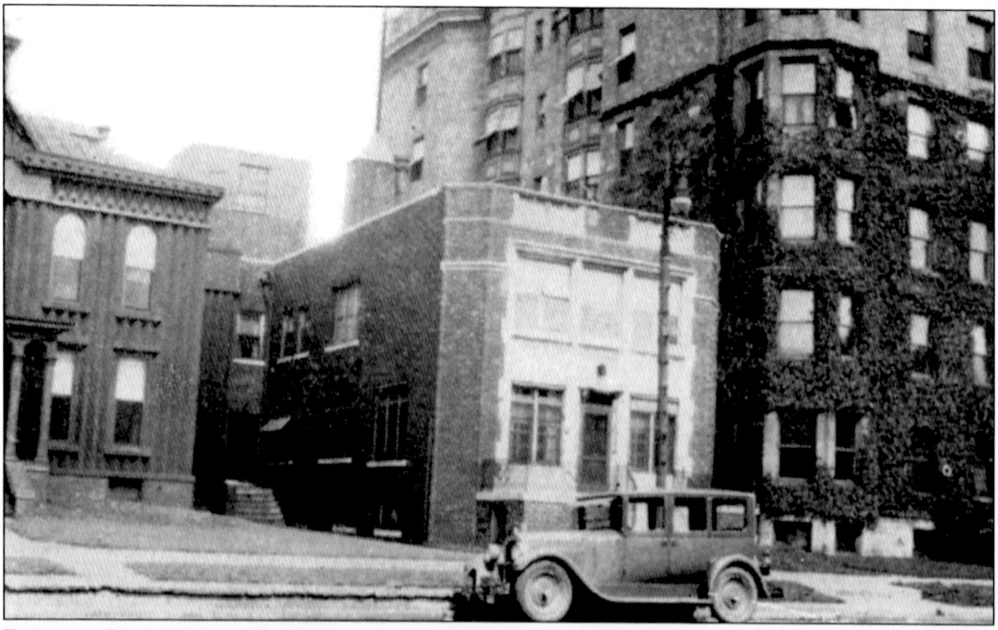

DETROIT DIAGNOSTIC HOSPITAL, c. 1927. A car is parked in front of this small hospital which was located at 995 E. Jefferson in Detroit. The hospital did diagnostic procedures only, and it was run by Miss Mary A. MacKay, R.N. It was later replaced by Jennings Hospital which was taken over by St. John's Riverview.

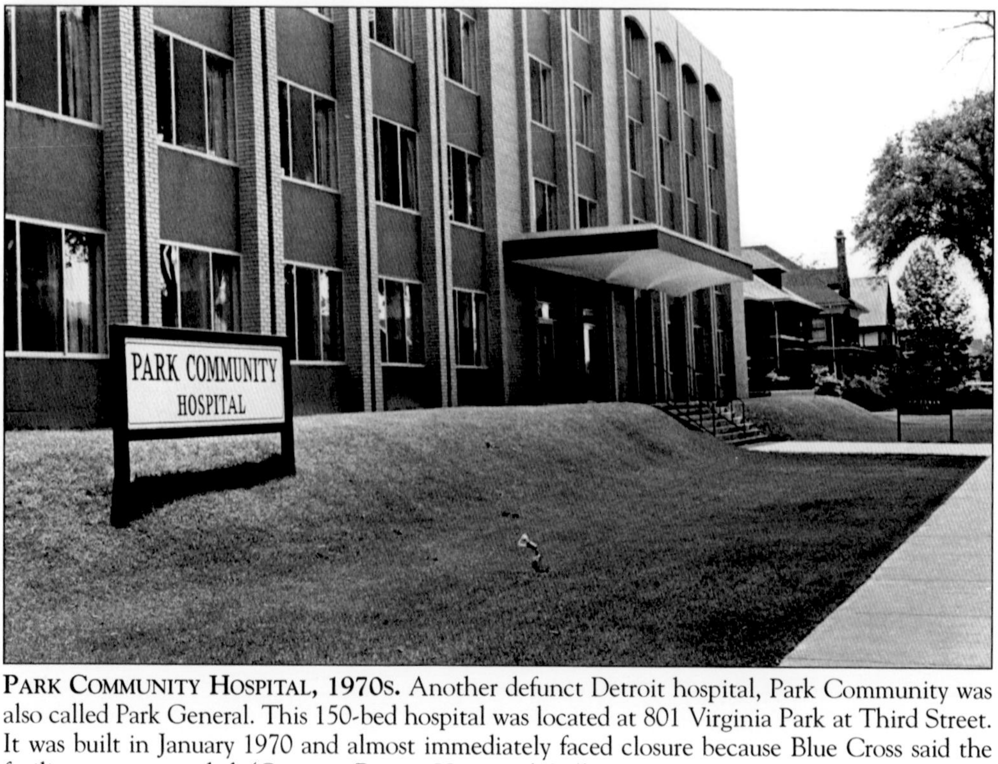

PARK COMMUNITY HOSPITAL, 1970S. Another defunct Detroit hospital, Park Community was also called Park General. This 150-bed hospital was located at 801 Virginia Park at Third Street. It was built in January 1970 and almost immediately faced closure because Blue Cross said the facility was not needed. (Courtesy Burton Historical Collection, Detroit Public Library.)

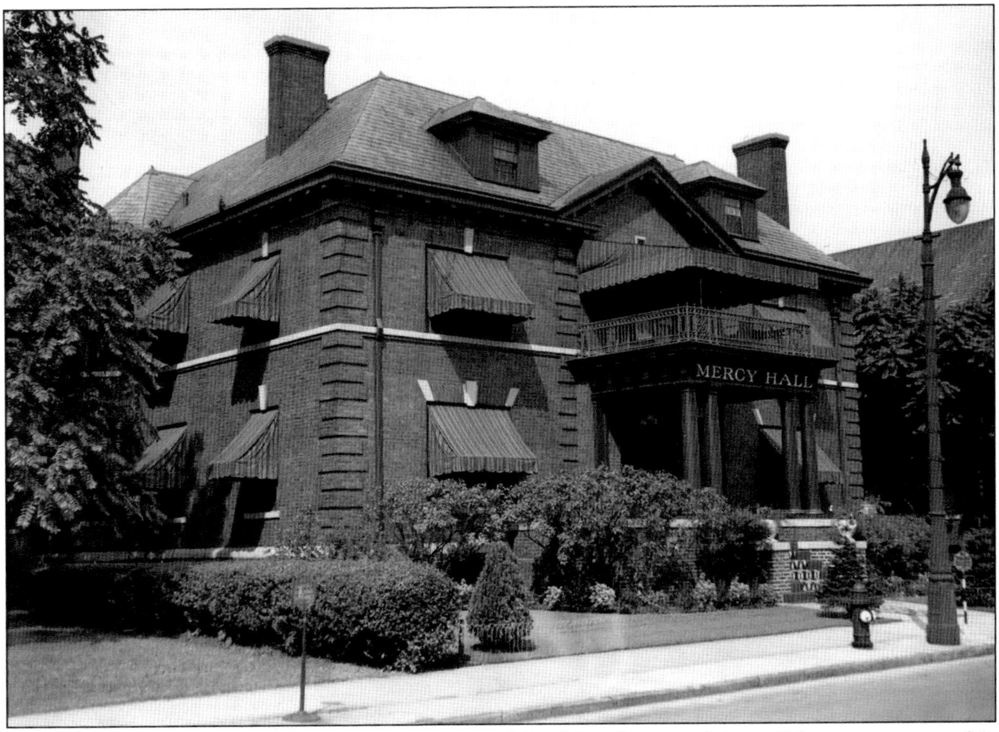

MERCY HALL HOSPITAL, c. 1940S. Organized by Miss Loretta Mary Gibson, a nurse, this facility was designed for the treatment of indigent cancer patients. Funding was provided by the Daughters of Charity. There were only six beds. It opened October 26, 1931. It was located at 269 Mack in Detroit. (Courtesy Burton Historical Collection, Detroit Public Library.)

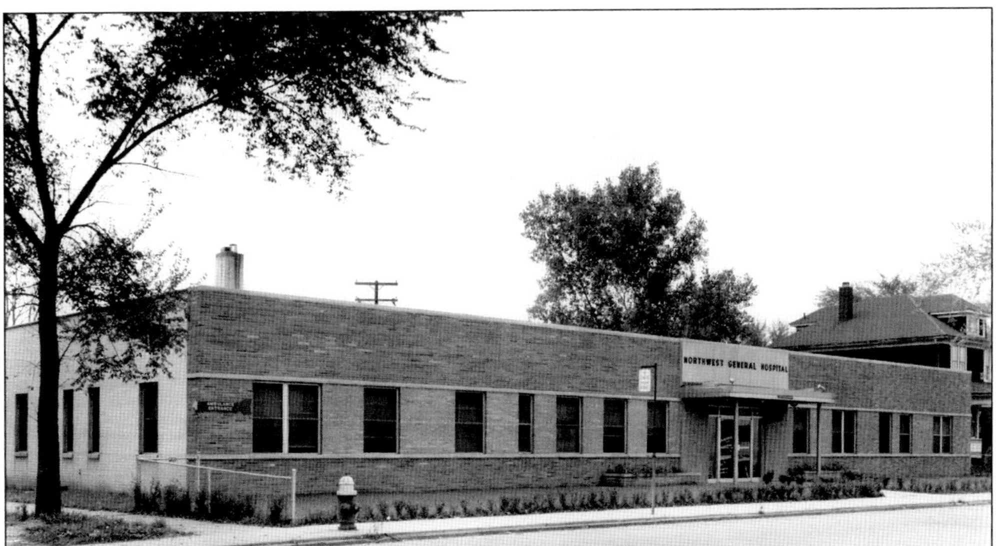

NORTHWEST GENERAL HOSPITAL. This 104-bed hospital at 8741 W. Chicago was built in 1953. In 1982 it became affiliated with Botsford General Hospital in Farmington Hills. It closed in 1990, another victim of declining Detroit population and changing health care needs. (Courtesy Burton Historical Collection, Detroit Public Library.)

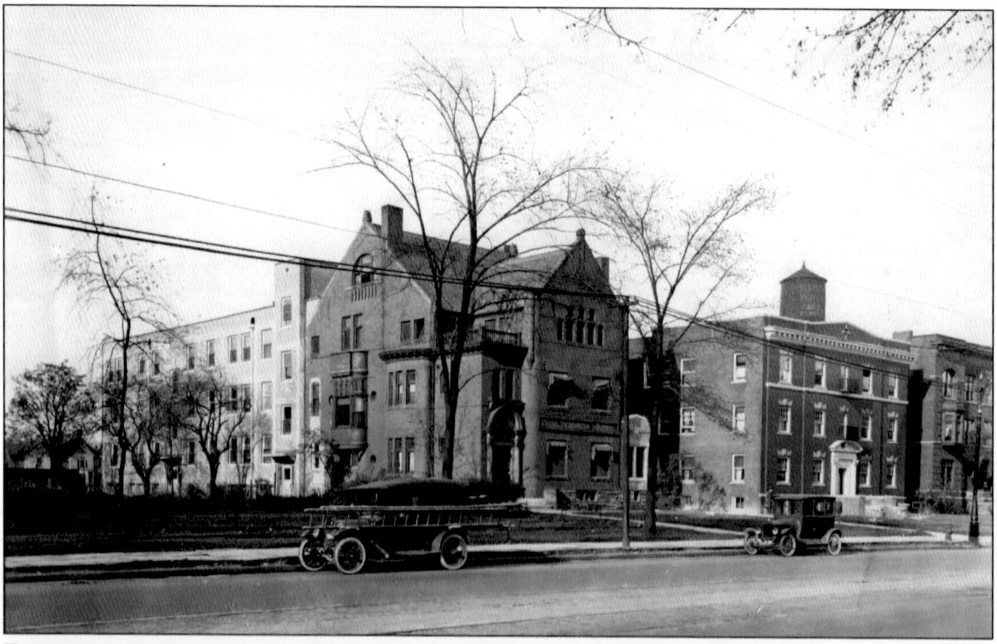

EVANGELICAL DEACONESS, 1921. Although this hospital only had 135 beds, it ran a training school for nurses. It was located at 3245 East Jefferson. It was run by the Deaconess order, a German Lutheran organization, that had hospitals in other states This hospital merged with St. Joseph Mercy in 1978 to form the Samaritan Health Center. Note the water tank of the King Motor Car Company. (Courtesy Burton Historical Collection, Detroit Public Library.)

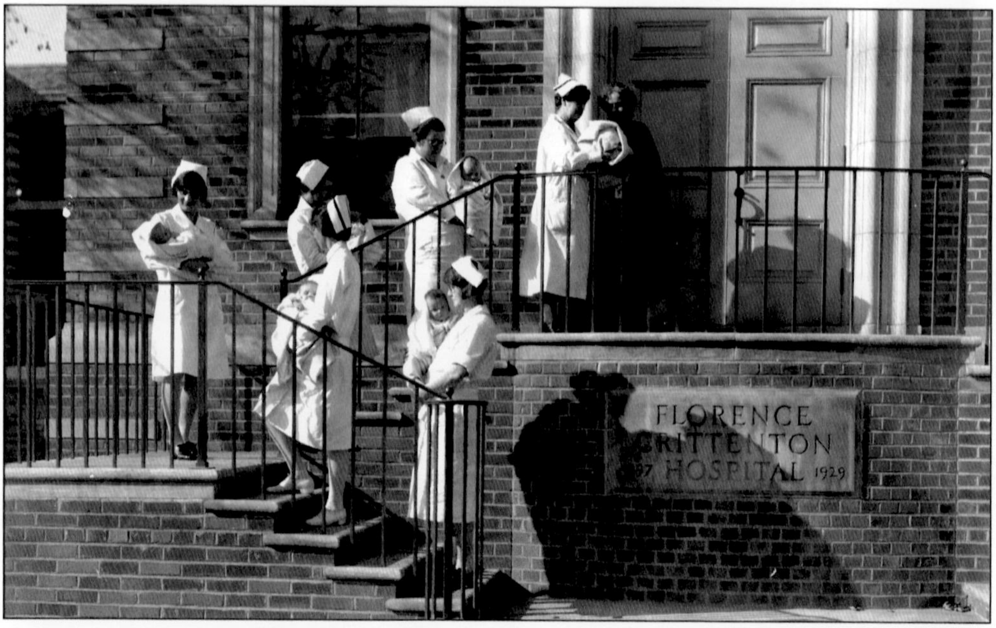

FLORENCE CRITTENTON HOSPITAL, 1965. A stream of nurses are carrying their little charges up the stairs into the building on E. Elizabeth Street in Detroit. Care was given to "unfortunate women and girls" and their babies. The hospital specialized in obstetrics, gynecology and pediatrics. It closed in 1976. (Courtesy Burton Historical Collection, Detroit Public Library.)

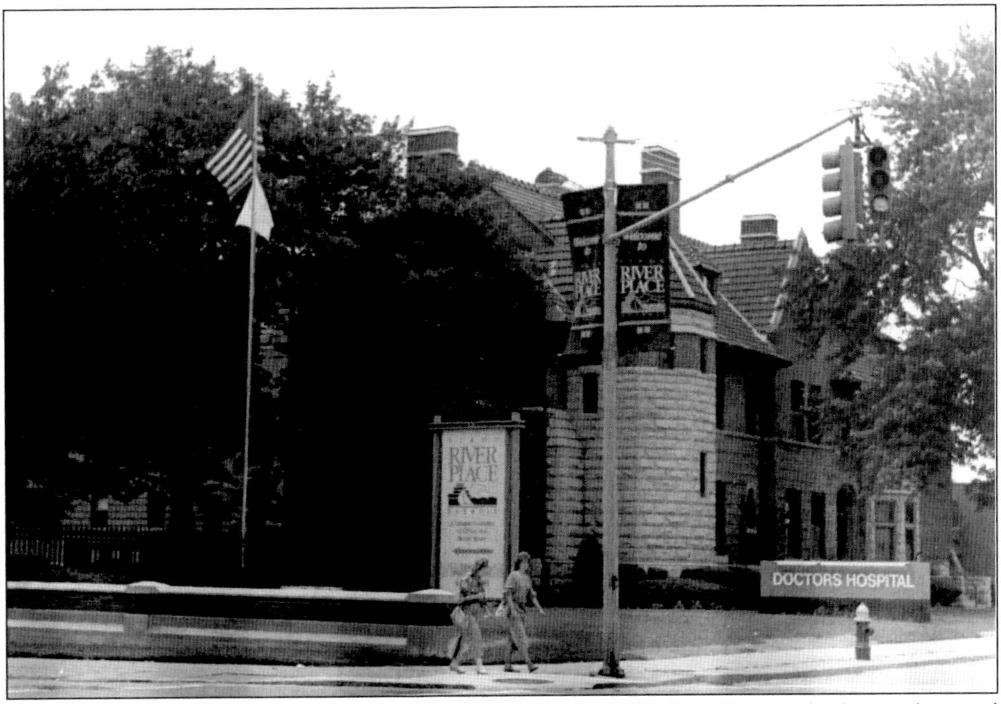

Doctor's Hospital. Originally this was the Franklin H. Walker House which was designed by Detroit architect George DeWitt Mason. Franklin H. Walker was a member of the Walker distillery family. The building is located at 2730 E. Jefferson, and it served as an industrial hospital until 1980. (Courtesy Burton Historical Collection, Detroit Public Library.)

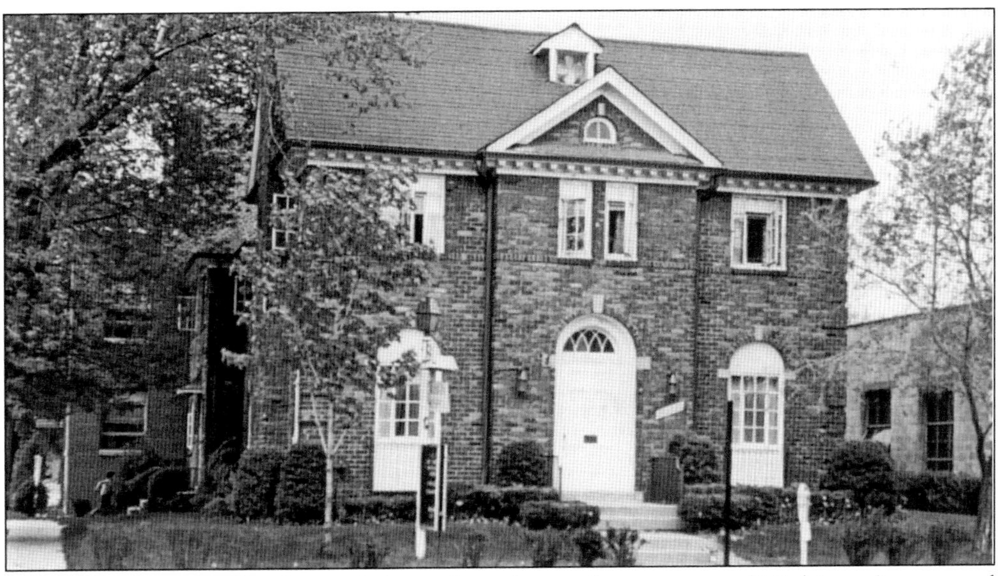

Nankin Hospital. This hospital, located on the northeast corner of Michigan Avenue and Sophia in Wayne, opened about 1931, and it was originally called the Caraway-Huff Clinic. It was owned by Dr. Archambeault. After the hospital closed, the building was used for efficiency apartments for a while. It was once a fine looking building as evidenced by this color postcard, but it now sits boarded up. (Courtesy Wayne Historical Museum.)

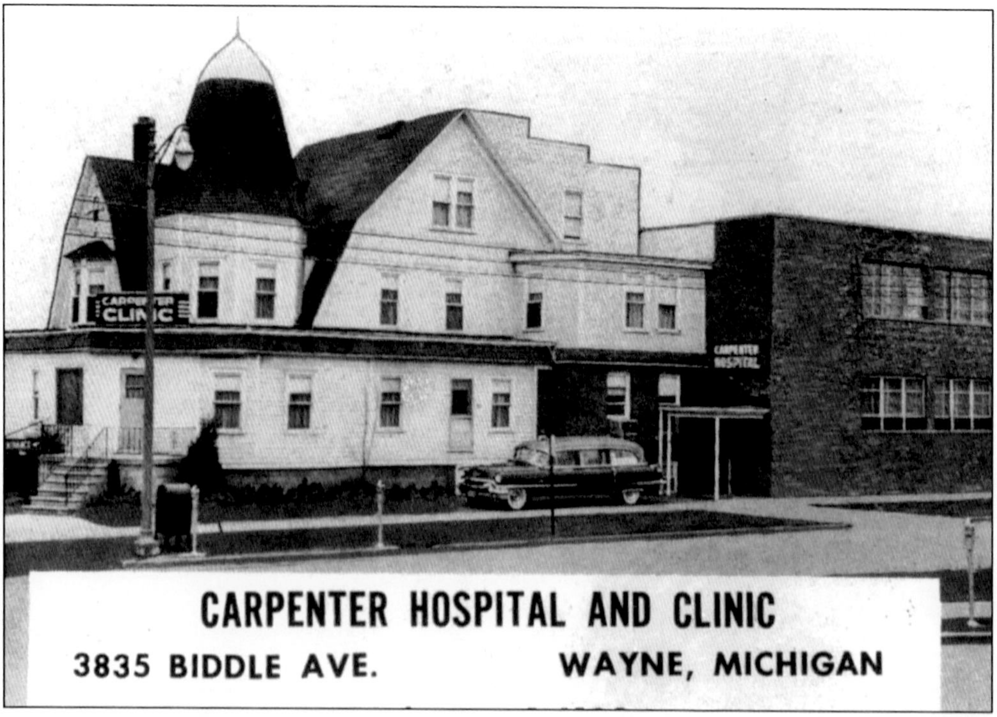

CARPENTER HOSPITAL AND CLINIC, 1960s. Dr. Clarence Carpenter founded this clinic and hospital in 1929, and it closed *c.* 1965. The reverse side of this postcard even had a map showing its location in Wayne, and listed all the services available, including sending a doctor to the scene of a severe accident. The Cadillac ambulance is parked and ready to go. (Courtesy Wayne Historical Museum.)

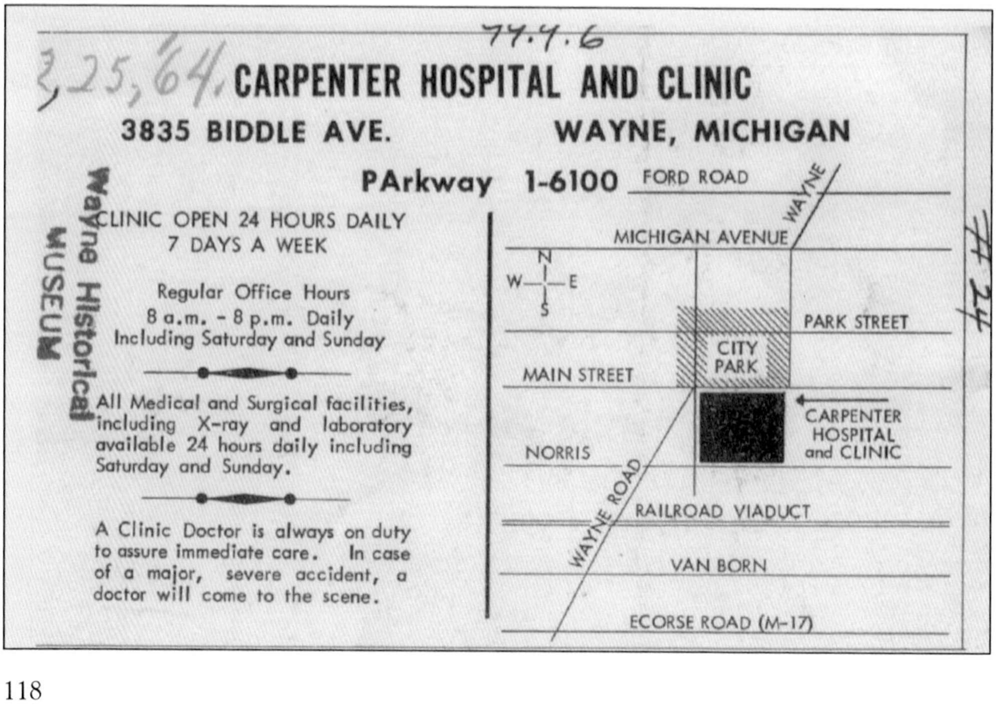

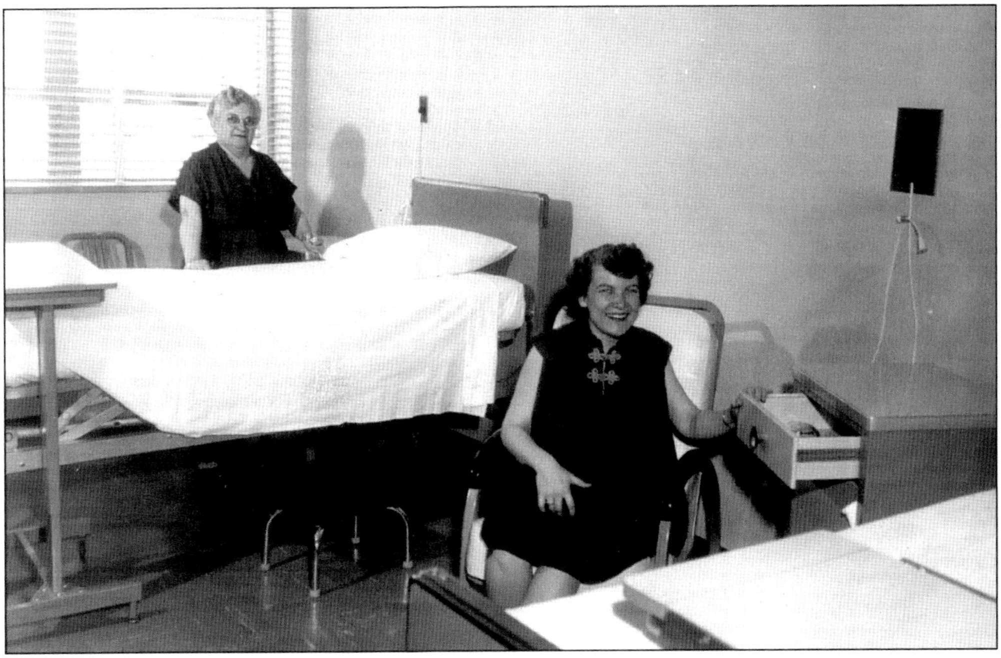

MATERNITY WARD, CARPENTER CLINIC, 1960S. A happy new mother poses in a typical patient room. The first child born at this Wayne hospital was the child of Tony Hill, a Melvindale policeman. The baby arrived in December of 1929. (Courtesy Wayne Historical Museum.)

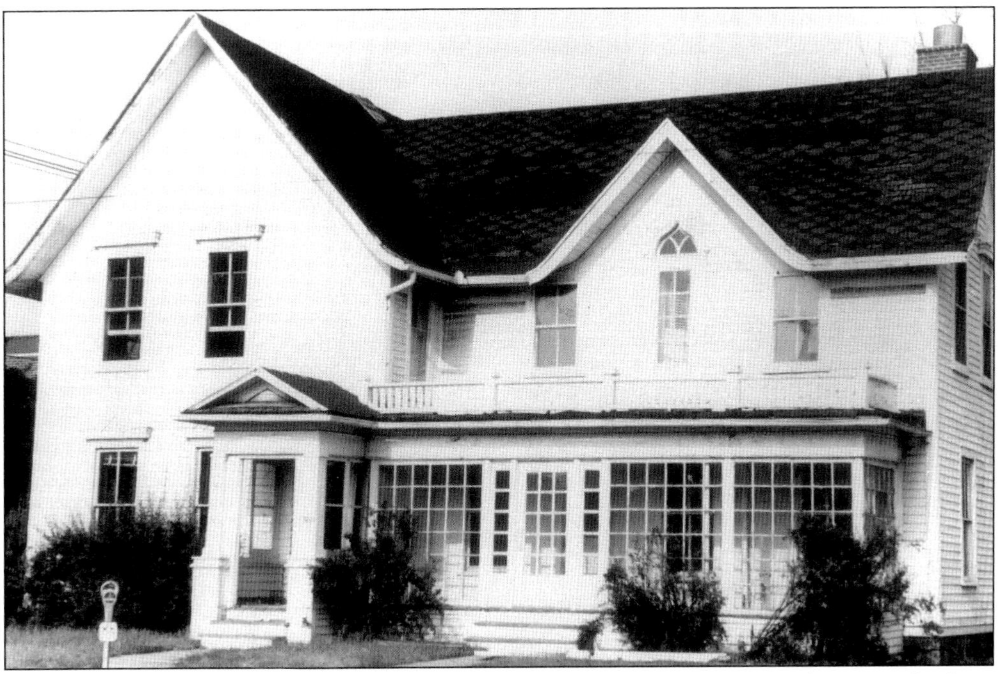

PARKER-VINCENT HOSPITAL, c. 1960. This old building was once the Pate house, and it later became a small hospital which was located on the west side of Washington between Park and Main streets directly north of the Congregational Church in Wayne. It is long gone due to urban renewal. (Courtesy Wayne Historical Museum.)

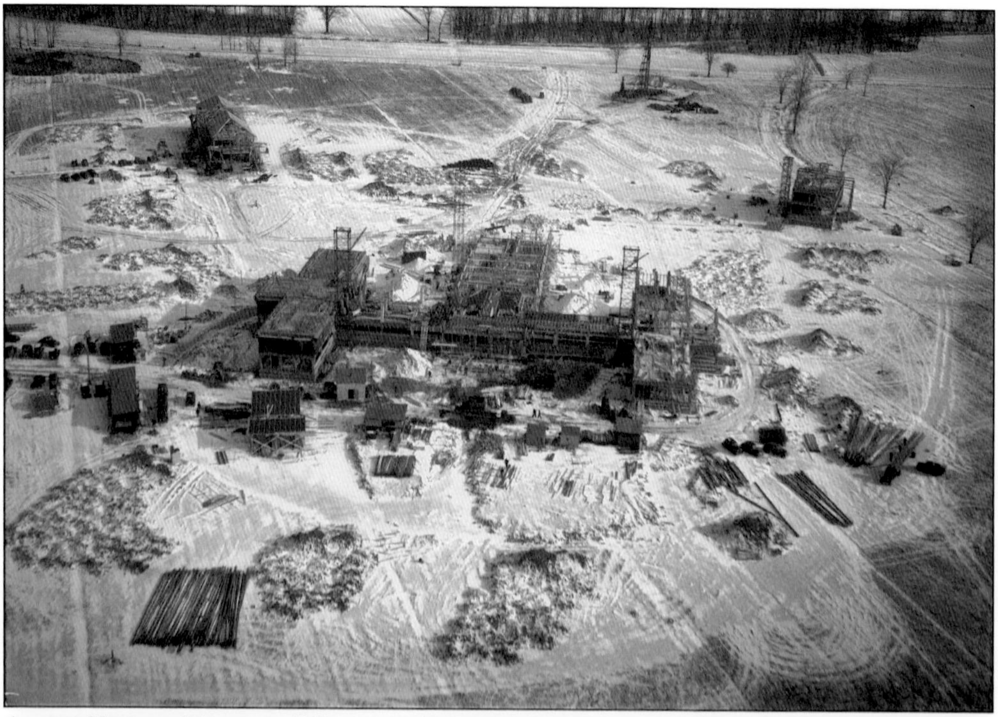

AERIAL VIEW OF VETERANS' HOSPITAL UNDER CONSTRUCTION, 1935. The U.S. government's 22-building treatment facility for disabled veterans opened in 1939 and closed in June of 1996 when a new facility opened in the Detroit Medical Center. The buildings were demolished in 2003, and the land reverted back to the Ford Motor Company. (Courtesy Walter P. Reuther Library, Wayne State University.)

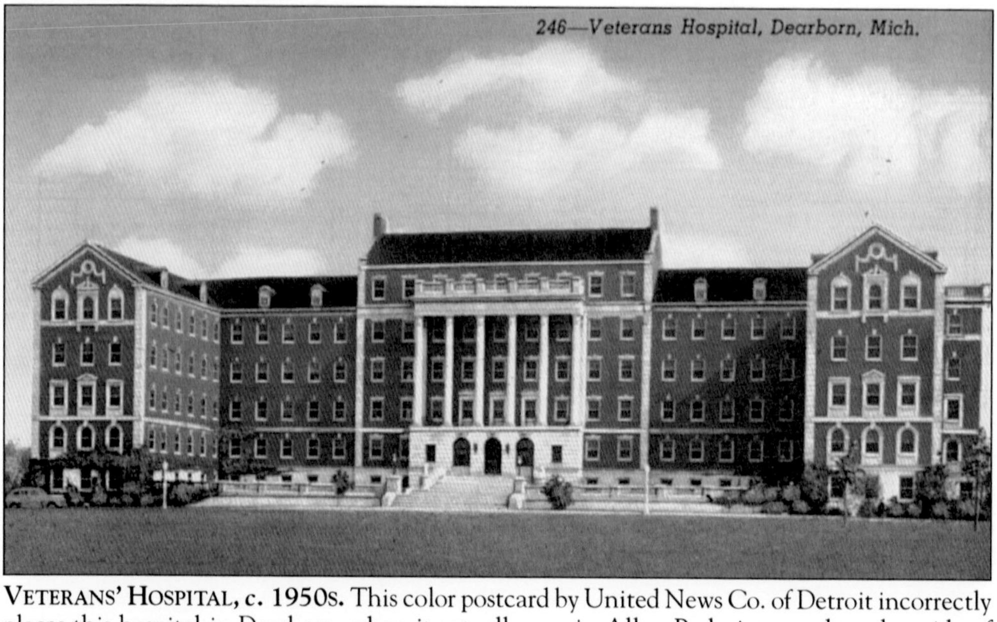

VETERANS' HOSPITAL, c. 1950S. This color postcard by United News Co. of Detroit incorrectly places this hospital in Dearborn, when it actually was in Allen Park, just on the other side of the Southfield Freeway which divides Dearborn and Allen Park.

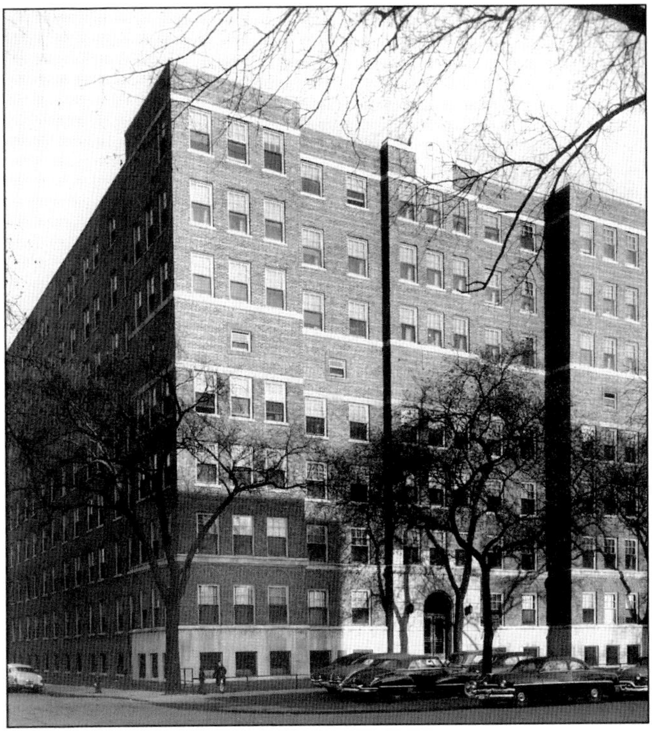

St. Joseph Mercy Hospital, Detroit, 1952. This 150-bed general hospital was located at 2200 East Grand Boulevard. It was built in 1925, and was run by the Sisters of Mercy. Before that, the sisters used the Samaritan hospital next door from 1922 until the new hospital was built. (Courtesy Sisters of Mercy Archives, Farmington, Michigan.)

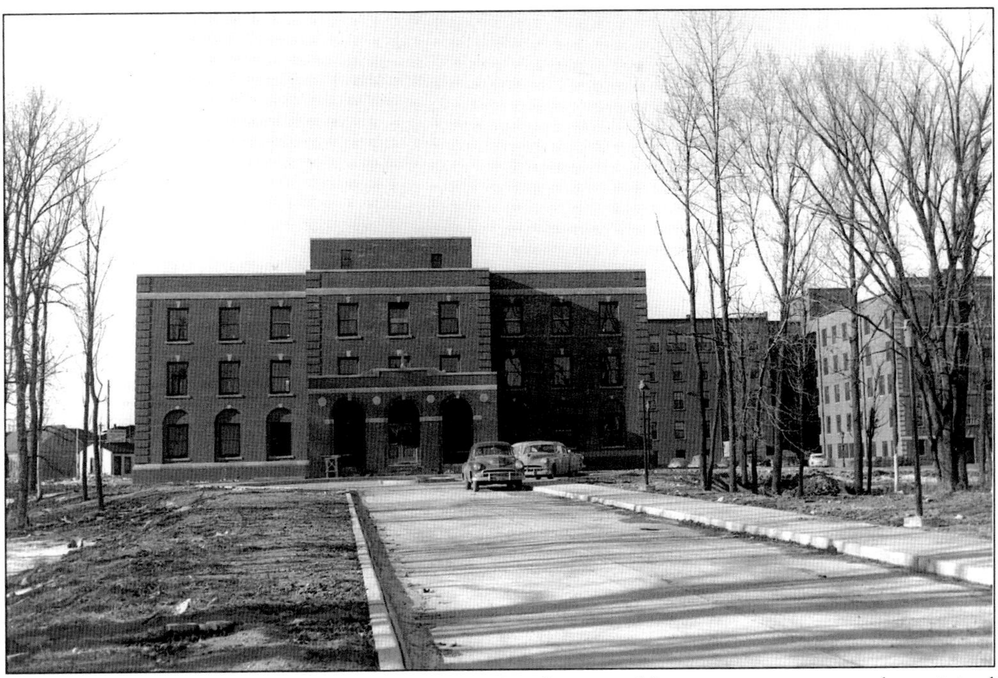

St. Joseph Mercy Hospital, Detroit, 1952. A new addition was put on to the original building which can be seen to the far right. This hospital merged with Evangelical Deaconess Hospital in 1978 to become the Samaritan Health Center. It was demolished in 1993 to make room for the General Motors Poletown plant. (Courtesy Walter P. Reuther Library, Wayne State University.)

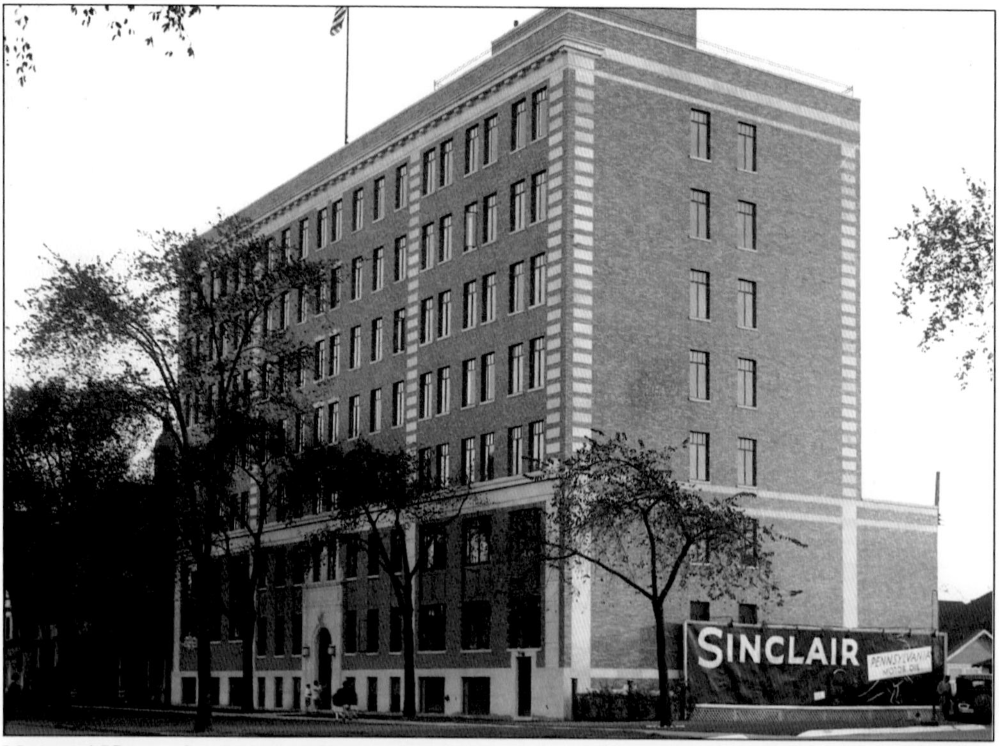

NURSES' HOME, ST. JOSEPH MERCY HOSPITAL, 1931. Nurses are seen entering the brand new nurses' home which was connected to the hospital on the other side of East Grand Boulevard by an underground tunnel. The nurses' home had a gymnasium, library, classrooms, and a cafeteria in the basement. There were accommodations for 135 nurses and sisters. (Courtesy Walter P. Reuther Library, Wayne State University.)

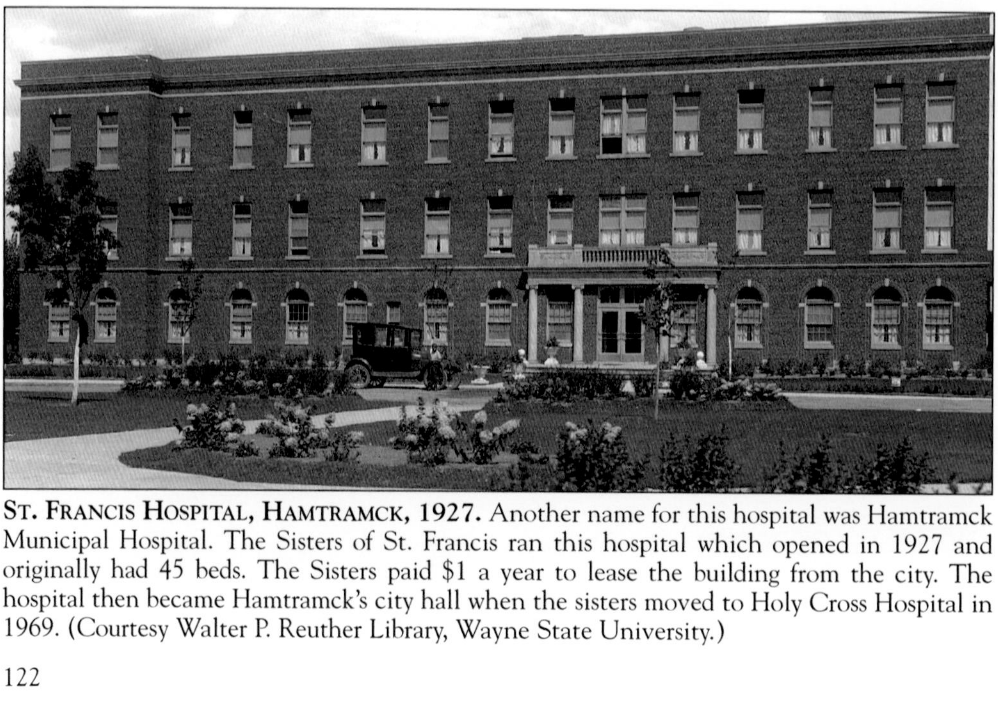

ST. FRANCIS HOSPITAL, HAMTRAMCK, 1927. Another name for this hospital was Hamtramck Municipal Hospital. The Sisters of St. Francis ran this hospital which opened in 1927 and originally had 45 beds. The Sisters paid $1 a year to lease the building from the city. The hospital then became Hamtramck's city hall when the sisters moved to Holy Cross Hospital in 1969. (Courtesy Walter P. Reuther Library, Wayne State University.)

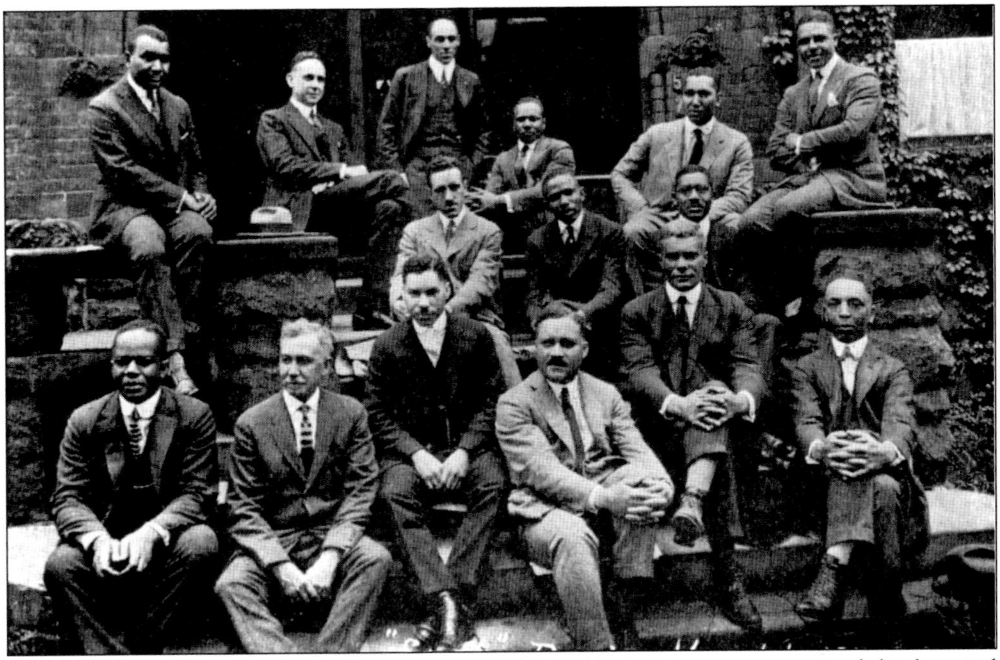

DUNBAR HOSPITAL, MEDICAL STAFF, 1922. Eighteen black doctors incorporated this hospital at 580 Frederick in 1918 as Detroit's first non-profit hospital for the black community. This hospital was later moved to Brush and Illinois and was renamed Parkside Hospital, and operated under that name until 1962. There is a historic marker on the site, which now houses an administrative headquarters and a museum. (Courtesy Burton Historical Collection, Detroit Public Library.)

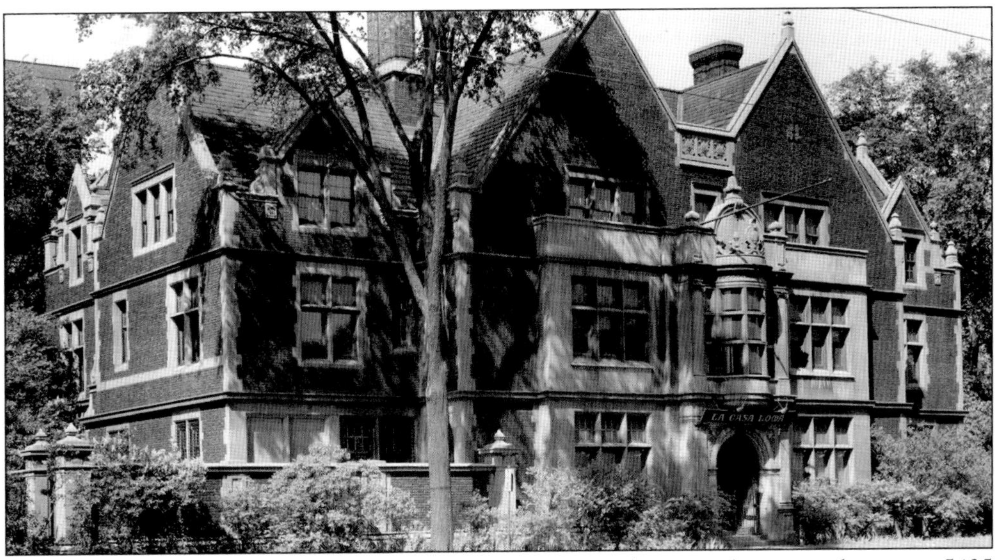

ART CENTRE HOSPITAL, 1942. The former Bowen residence and carriage house at 5435 Woodward, opposite the Wardell Hotel on Kirby, was remodeled into Art Centre Hospital. This osteopathic hospital had 75 beds, and the x-ray and laboratory facilities were behind the main building. It later merged with Zeigler Osteopathic Hospital. (Courtesy Burton Historical Collection, Detroit Public Library.)

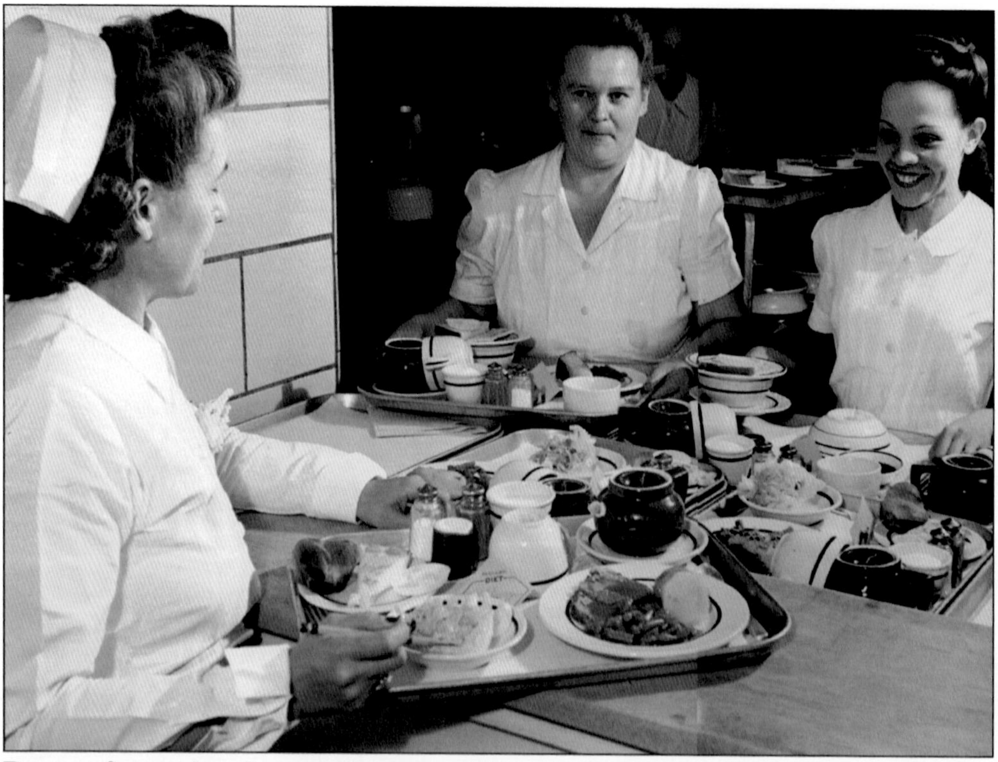

DIETARY STAFF, ART CENTRE HOSPITAL, 1942. This food looks a lot more appetizing than what one would get in a hospital today. With only 75 patients to cook for, special attention could be paid to meals. (Courtesy Burton Historical Collection, Detroit Public Library.)

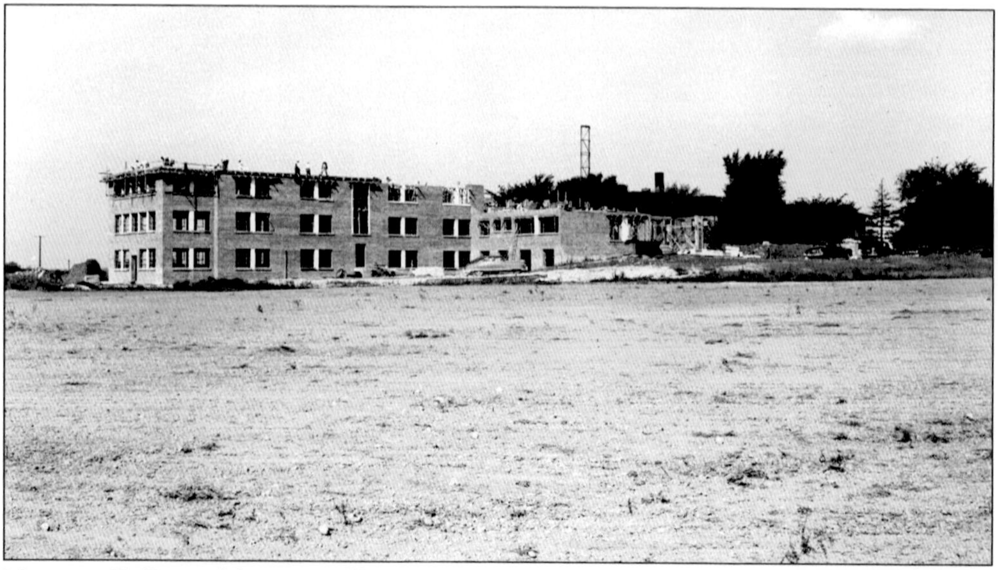

MARTHA T. BERRY MEMORIAL HOSPITAL, MOUNT CLEMENS, 1949. This photo shows the hospital under construction. It opened in 1950 and was named as a memorial to the wife of Dr. Henry G. Berry (1865–1945), a Macomb County physician. It was run by Macomb County. (Courtesy the *Macomb Daily*.)

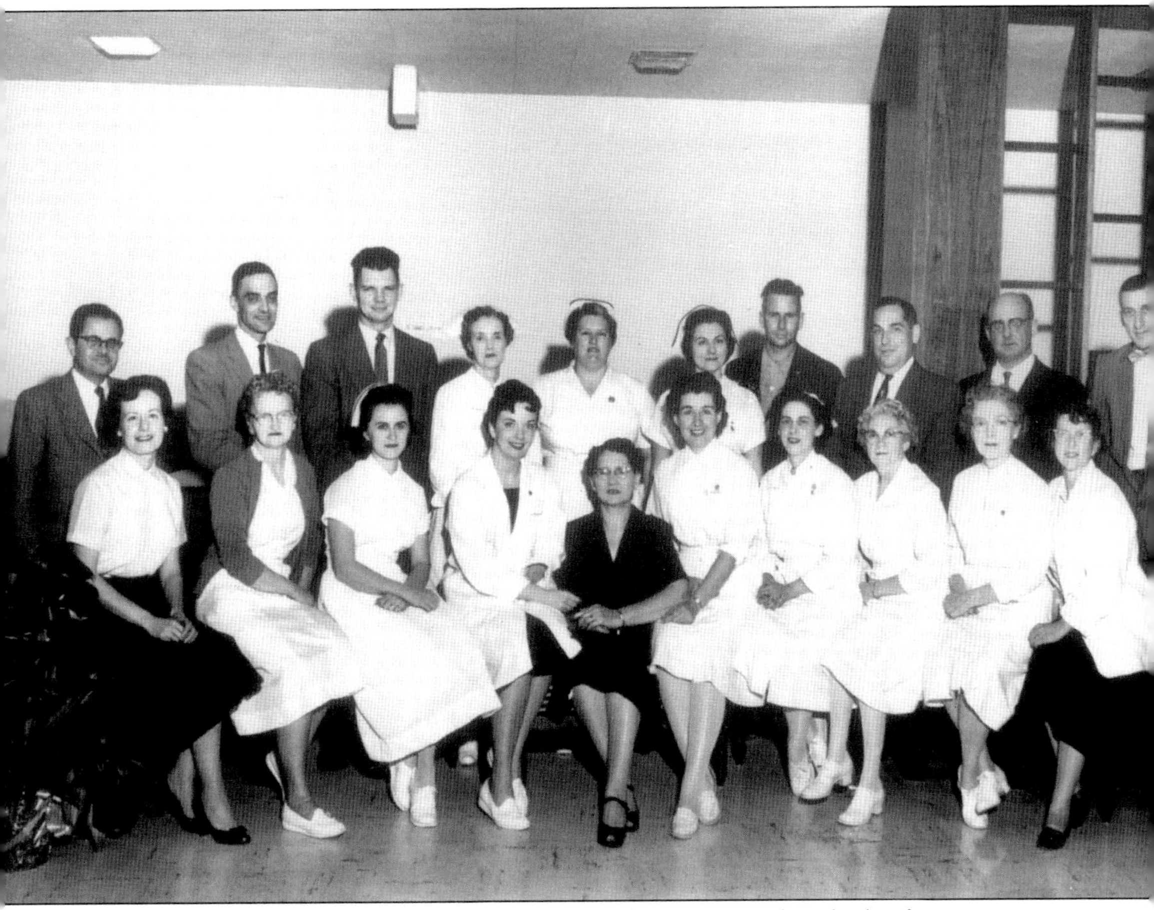

STAFF OF ANNAPOLIS HOSPITAL, 1957. Staff members are posed with the first patient at the Annapolis Unit of The Peoples Community Hospital Authority (PCHA). Pictured here are, from left to right: (front row) Miss H. Theakes, Medical Records; Mrs. O. McClinton, Housekeeping; Mrs. G. Yonish, Recovery Room; Mrs. M. Van Gilder, Laboratory; the patient Mrs. Clejo Brandon; Miss R. McQuade, Dietary; Mrs. M. Surgenor, Director of Nurses; Miss I. Baker, Obstetrics; Mrs. M. Gariepy, Anesthesia; and Dr. Engstrom, Pathology. In the second row are Arthur C. Forche, Superintendent; R. Schlief, Purchasing; Neil Caldwell, Pharmacy; Mrs. V. Gilmore, Emergency Room; Mrs. I. Creech, Central Supply; Mrs. Elaine Hanson, Operating Room; W. O'Neal, Maintenance; J. Hulme, Business Office; Dr. Rekshan, Radiology; and W. Barret, Laundry. This photo appeared in the *Wayne Eagle* November 14, 1957. The Michigan State Legislature repealed the PCHA in 1988, and all the former PCHA hospitals became part of the Oakwood Healthcare System. (Courtesy Wayne Historical Museum.)

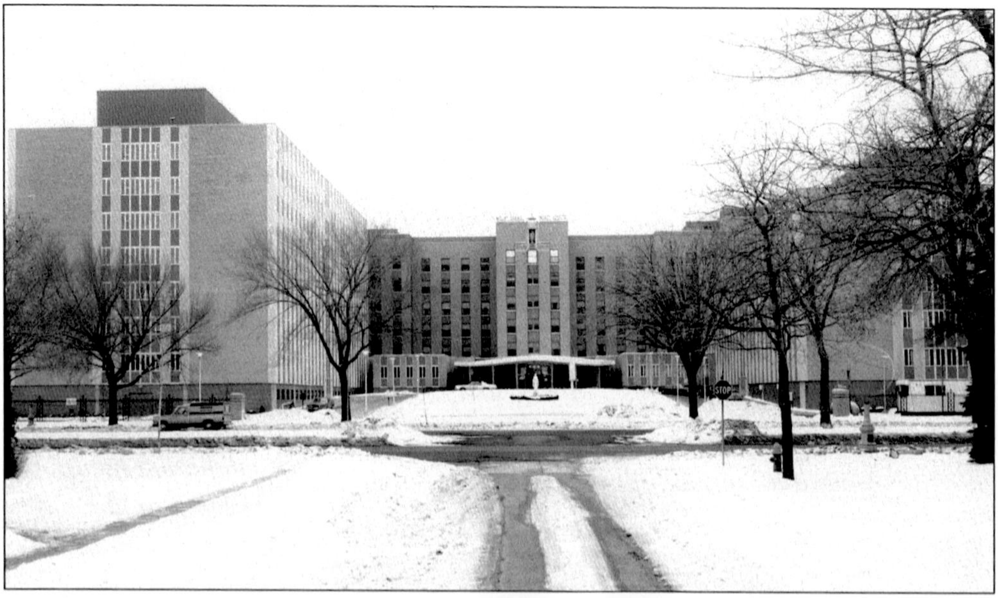

MT. CARMEL MERCY HOSPITAL, 1960S. Shown here on a wintry day is another major Detroit general hospital which was run by the Sisters of Mercy. It was built in 1939 and located at 6701 W. Outer Drive. At one time it had 560 beds and 1,800 employees. This hospital merged with Grace Hospital in 1991. (Courtesy Sisters of Mercy Archives, Farmington, Michigan.)

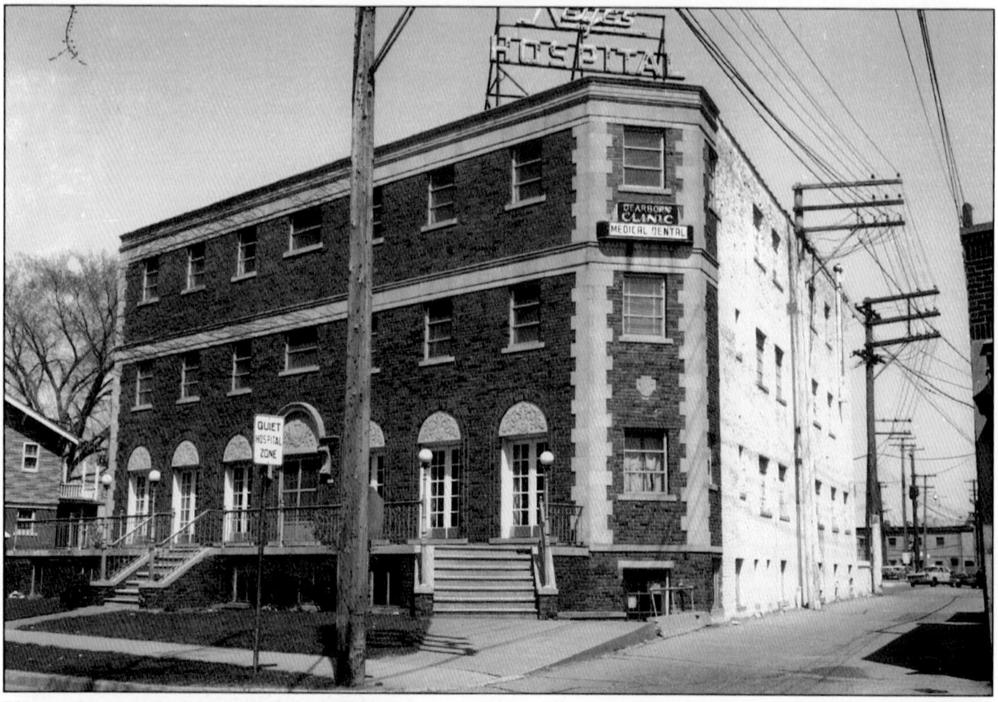

KEYES DEARBORN DIAGNOSTIC HOSPITAL, 1960S. This small hospital was opened in 1932 by Eugene C. Keyes, who was first a dentist, and then became a physician and surgeon. It was located at Maple, north of the Dearborn City Hall, and had 65 adult beds and 30 bassinets. The building was leveled in 1965 and the site became a parking lot. (Courtesy Dearborn Historical Museum.)

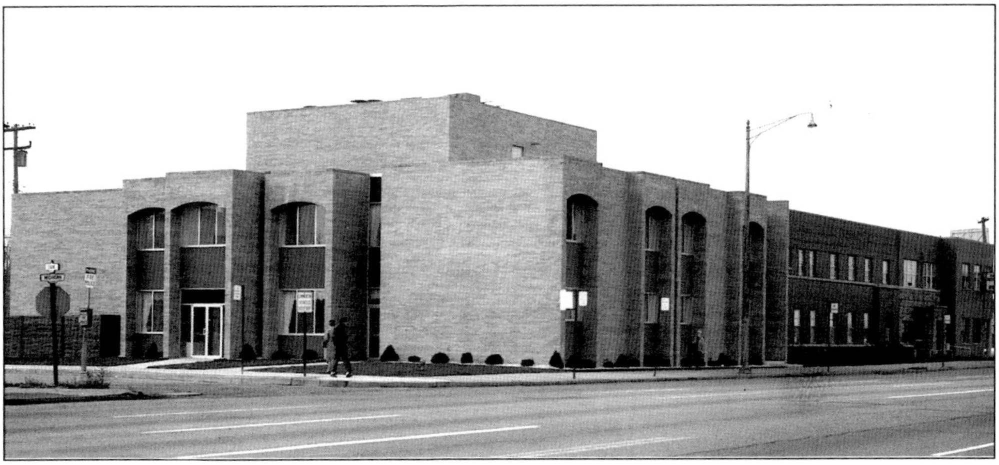

DEARBORN MEDICAL CENTER, c. 1970S. Now absorbed into the large Oakwood Health System, this hospital was once a private hospital which opened about 1950 at 10149–10151 Michigan Avenue two blocks west of Wyoming. It was used as an industrial clinic for several years after it was no longer used as a hospital. (Courtesy Dearborn Historical Museum.)

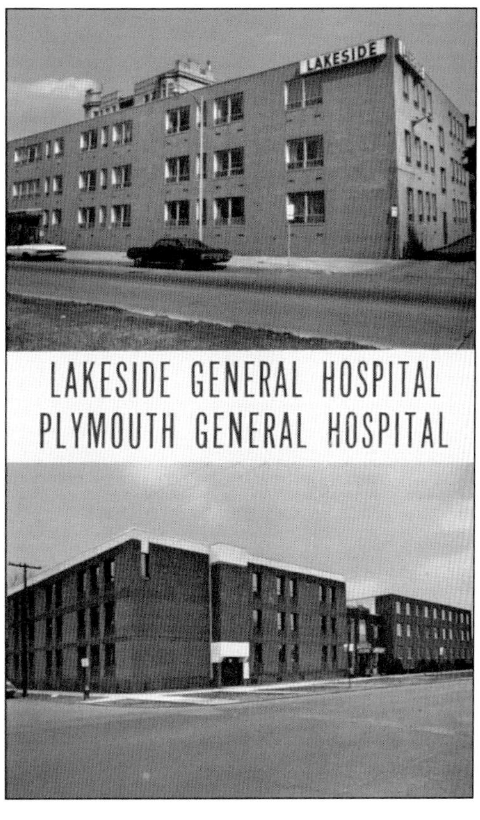

LAKESIDE GENERAL/PLYMOUTH GENERAL HOSPITALS, 1970S. Two of many small Detroit hospitals, Lakeside was located at 988 E. Larned Boulevard and Plymouth was located at 15361 Plymouth Road. Lakeside opened in 1945, and Plymouth in 1952. Both were operated by the Greater Detroit Community Hospitals, Inc. and are shown together on a postcard.

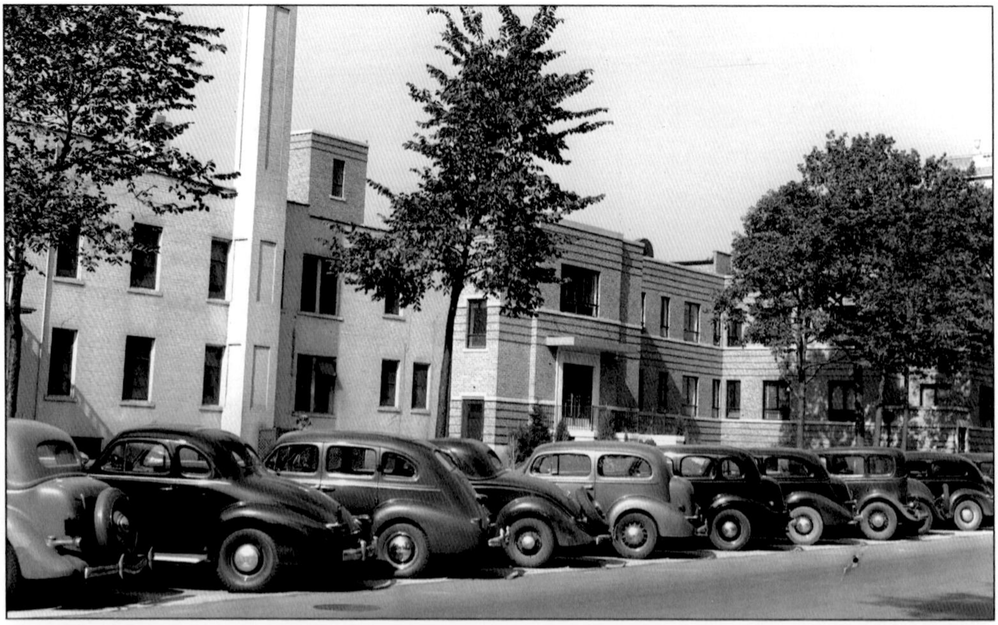

Detroit Osteopathic Hospital, 1937. This hospital was located at Third and Highland in Highland Park, and it was Michigan's first osteopathic hospital. It was built in bits and pieces starting in 1919. Team doctors for the Detroit Lions, Tigers, Pistons, and Red Wings were staff members. It closed in 1992, and was purchased by St. John Detroit Riverview Hospital. (Courtesy Walter P. Reuther Library, Wayne State University.)

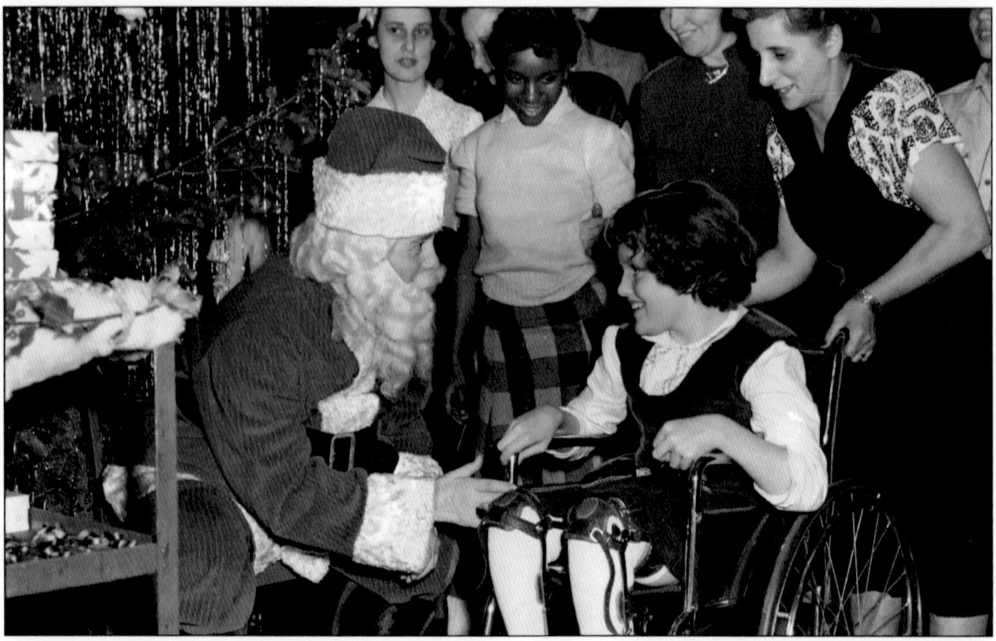

Patients from Detroit Orthopedic Clinic, 1950s. Santa Claus lends an attentive ear to Sally Farney, age ten, at a Christmas party given by the Briggs Girls Club. Sally was one of 66 guests from the Detroit Orthopedic Clinic. The party was held at the Outer Drive plant of Briggs Manufacturing Company. (Courtesy Burton Historical Collection, Detroit Public Library.)